Medical
KNOWLEDGE
for fun

To Paul

Medical
KNOWLEDGE
for fun

Richard Worcester

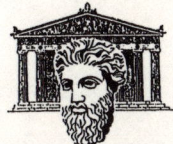

The Parthenon Publishing Group
International Publishers in Medicine, Science & Technology

NEW YORK   LONDON

Published in the UK and Europe by
The Parthenon Publishing Group Limited,
Casterton Hall, Carnforth,
Lancs. LA6 2LA, England

Published in the USA by
The Parthenon Publishing Group Inc.,
One Blue Hill Plaza,
PO Box 1564, Pearl River,
New York 10965, USA

British Library Cataloguing in Publication Data

Worcester, Richard
    Medical knowledge for fun
    I. Title
    610. 76

ISBN 1-85070-685-9

Library of Congress Cataloging-in-Publication Data

Worcester, Richard
    Medical Knowledge for Fun / Richard Worcester
        p.   cm.
    ISBN 1-85070-685-9
        1. Medicine--Miscellanea.   I. Title.
R706.W67 1995
610--dc20   95-34795
                                                                          CIP

Printed and bound by Bookcraft (Bath) Ltd., Midsomer Norton

Contents

About the Author

*Richard Worcester is a pseudonym which conceals the identity of a
distinguished Oxford professor. His remarkable and all-embracing knowledge of the classics,
modern languages and science – no less than the detailed field of medicine – has subscribed to the writing
and contents of this fascinating book. His professional life continues in the practice and teaching of
medicine. He is an Honorary Fellow of his college, where his rooms have been named after him.
His engaging sense of humour readily pervades the text and his concern
for the imparting of knowledge is also evident throughout.*

Introduction

Medicine has a long life and a long history. It is as old as mankind itself. Its branches permeate all aspects of human existence and so much of its history and evolution is of the greatest interest. We are all better informed for this knowledge and obtaining it, if approached in the right way, can be the most rewarding fun. This book has been written in a light-hearted fashion to impart the maximum number of facts with the minimum amount of effort. It is hoped that you will enjoy it and make good use of what you learn. Although light-hearted this book deals with life – both the present and the past. In a few instances it touches upon death – that final remedy to which each one of us is heir. Medical knowledge knows no boundaries; it is truly international. To the benefit of mankind its progress and discoveries are freely made to the world in attempts to serve and alleviate human disease and suffering.

Yet it is remarkable how, in the world today, medical knowledge – and pseudo-knowledge – have become such striking news. We are subjected to a daily barrage from newspapers, magazines, radio and television – and even coffee-table gossip. The media of communication vie with each other for dramatic articles, features and programmes each covering the more sensational aspects of human suffering and its cures. If we so wish, from the comfort of our armchairs at home and with the flick of a switch, we can now watch the most gory details of major surgical operations or view lifelike and most realistic pro-grammes of activity in casualty departments, simulated by actors for entertainment and enjoyment. Medical terminology is bandied about – quite often inappropriately – in many areas of everyday speech. Oneupmanship in this particular activity finds a ready rôle and is rife.

Does this dramatization serve any useful purpose other than satisfying a morose curiosity and need for morbid entertainment? An increased awareness of health and disease can only be a good thing. But if matters become out of control we are merely in danger of producing a nation of hypochondriacs. 'Fitness freaks', 'food freaks' and 'health freaks' are now only too well established and breed by a process of contagion. If knowledge engenders fear, worry and irrational guilt no useful purpose is served and we find that many of the half-truths suggested merely debase the quality of life and cause anxiety on a major scale.

Fear and false suggestions promote flights into bizzare so-called 'therapies'. Here the world of commerce obligingly steps in and multi-million pound industries will persuade you to look younger, look thinner, enjoy greater joie de vivre or live longer, capitalizing on anxieties subtly induced.

Genetic endowment – the gift from our fore-bears – is reponsible for so much that makes up our lives and, like it or not, the action of these genes will predominate in spite of egocentric efforts to modify ourselves according to the dictates of trend or fashion.

To have had the opportunity to study medicine,

together with its resulting opportunity for service to one's fellow creatures, has been – in the author's opinion – one of life's greatest privileges. A vast accumulation of knowledge and experience since time immemorial has been handed down and temporarily entrusted to the modern doctor. Today, that knowledge is increasing and expanding with breathtaking rapidity and it is mind-boggling to speculate the advances a further ten years will witness.

The quizzes of this book embrace a very wide field. Don't worry if a number of questions stump you – merely look up the answers and learn from them. Each quiz is framed for your enjoyment. The acquisition of knowledge in such an interesting field can only be one of considerable pleasure.

Lastly, I wish to thank all my friends who so kindly encouraged the production of this small volume. In particular, I wish to acknowledge with very great gratitude the most helpful and courteous assistance of Miss Julia Hamer-Hunt who revealed to me the hidden powers of the computer and who prepared the manuscript so swiftly and so expertly. Her inspiration throughout would be difficult in any way to overestimate.

Richard Worcester
Oxford

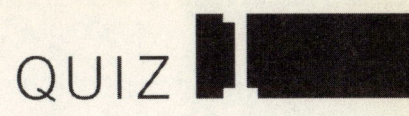

Think of a number

Some numbers are lucky – others are not. There are mystic numbers, magic numbers, round numbers and odd numbers. They can be significant to a statistician or sinister to the superstitious. In some cases, the number may well be up.

You can prove anything with figures; but can you say what the following numbers suggest in the field of medicine?

1 98.4

2 32

3 120/80

4 99

5 606

6 9.3

7 280

8 46

9 6/6

10 72

answers overleaf

1 Body temperature Normal body temperature is 98.4 degrees Fahrenheit when measured in the mouth. Even so, our temperatures vary slightly in health. They are usually lower in the morning and higher in the evening, and differ by an interval of approximately one degree. The metric equivalent of normal body temperature is 37 degrees Celsius.

2 Adult teeth There are 32 teeth in the full set of an adult. The upper and lower jaws each bear four incisor or cutting teeth, two canine or eye teeth, four premolar and six molar teeth. The premolars and molars are grinding teeth, and the last molars to erupt are the so-called 'wisdom teeth'.

3 Blood pressure Our blood pressure normally varies within quite wide limits and depends on what is being done at any given moment. The fraction 120/80 records the standard value for an adult at rest. 120 millimetres of mercury is the pressure on contraction of the heart; 80 millimetres is the pressure on relaxation.

4 Chest examination Ninety-nine is the number you are asked to say during an examination of your chest. Its sound carries well through the chest wall and can be heard with a stethoscope. Its vibrations are felt with the hand. These qualities change when the chest is diseased.

5 Salvarsan Salvarsan was the name Paul Ehrlich gave to his substance Number 606. After experimenting with hundreds of different compounds, he found in substance Number 606 a remedy for syphilis which made medical history in the year 1909. Salvarsan is an organic compund of arsenic, chemically known as arsphenamine.

6 Calorie value per gramme of fat Each gramme of fat burnt by the body yields 9.3 calories of energy. This, by contrast, is more than twice the energy value obtained from burning an equivalent mass of either carbohydrate or protein. Fat, therefore, is our most concentrated way of storing energy. Our fat reserves supply calories when times are hard.

7 Duration of pregnancy The figure 280 is taken as the number of days to a normal pregnancy, but individual variations are frequent. If the first day of the last menstrual period is noted, the expected date of delivery can be calculated by adding nine months and nine days.

8 Body cell chromosomes Each body cell contains 46 chromosomes. Chromosomes carry genes which confer the characteristics we have inheritied from our parents. In contrast, the germ cells contain only half this number. This means that the new cell formed at fertilization will again bear the full quota of 46 chromosomes.

9 Normal sight Sight is tested at a distance of 6 metres and the smallest letters on the optician's card should be read. Such normal sight is written as 6/6 for each eye. Degrees of short sightedness are expressed by a change in the numerator (the distance from the card needed to read the letters) of this fraction and could be written as, for example, 3/6.

10 Pulse rate The standard average pulse rate at rest is taken as 72 beats per minute. Quite wide variations, however, can be met in normal health. Emotion, exercise or fever all accelerate the pulse. Children have more rapid pulses, but in athletes the rate is slow and may only register 50 beats per minute.

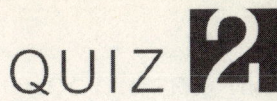

Myth and medicine

Greek and Roman influence in healing is traditional. Signs of their ancient practice have survived the centuries and persist today in many forms. The answers to the clues here illustrate how classical mythology still serves modern medicine.

1 The cares of the world rest on this bone in the neck.

2 A wide-eyed Fate with a dry mouth?

3 The God of Medicine.

4 Was cleanliness next to her godliness?

5 Not washing his tendon proved fatal.

6 His royal tragedy became a complex for psycho-analysts.

7 A mortified Greek maiden who spun this membrane of the brain?

8 The shepherd who gave his name to this unpleasant disease.

9 Sometimes considered the God of Surgery.

10 Her head on the abdomen might well petrify.

answers overleaf

1 Atlas This Titan helped wage war against Zeus, and in defeat was condemned to carry the heavens upon his shoulders. The first cervical vertebra carries the skull in a similar manner, and for this reason bears the same name.

2 Atropos Atropos was one of the three Fates and held the shears to cut the thread of life. The drug atropine is named after her. Atropine dilates the pupil and dries the mouth, and is found in the plant deadly nightshade *Atropa belladonna*. It is of great use in ophthalmology and in anaesthetics.

3 Aesculapius This god had his own special temples throughout Greece. So miraculous and so many were his cures that Zeus, fearing that men might cheat death altogether, destroyed Aesculapius with a thunderbolt. The serpent, which was sacred to him, is seen today in many medical emblems.

4 Hygeia Hygeia was the Goddess of Health and is often seen in ancient art feeding a snake from a cup. Hygiene, the branch of medicine dealing with the prevention of disease, is named after her. Preventing disease is preferable to all the spectacular cures.

5 Achilles In infancy, this hero was plunged into the river Styx. Its waters rendered him invulnerable wherever they washed him. The heel by which he was held remained dry, and an arrow piercing him here killed him. In our bodies, the Achilles' tendon can be felt just above the back of the heel.

6 Oedipus This King of Thebes unwittingly killed his father and wed his own mother as had been prophesied by the oracle. He freed his land from the terror of the Sphinx by solving her riddle. The Oedipus complex of the psychoanalysts denotes attitudes which may develop in a child towards its parents.

7 Arachne This skilful maiden challenged the goddess Minerva to a spinning contest. In Arachne's chagrin at losing, she attempted suicide by hanging but was turned into a spider which hung from its thread of silk. The arachnoid membrane is the middle of the three cerebral meninges and is named after its cobweb appearance.

8 Syphilis This was the name of a shepherd in the classic poem by Frascatorius in 1530. This poem describes accurately the disease sent by the gods to the shepherd for invoking their wrath, and which now bears his name. Before this, syphilis was known as the Great Pox or French Disease.

9 Chiron This wise and cultured Centaur, half man half horse, taught surgery to the Greek heroes. At that time, surgery comprised largely the removal of spear and arrow-heads and the dressing of wounds with medicinal herbs. Chiron is seen in the heavens as the constellation Sagittarius, ninth sign of the zodiac.

10 Medusa This Gorgon had hair of serpents and turned to stone all who looked on her. Rarely, the superficial veins of the anterior abdominal wall swell and become varicose. Their snake-like appearance as they radiate from the navel has led this condition to be called 'Medusa's Head'.

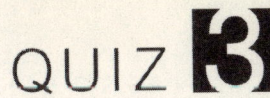

Old wives' tales

The answers to this quiz are well known but quite untrue. With the clues here, they form a collection of widely held fallacies. Most have been handed down for generations as old wives' tales, which no one seems to have thought of bringing up to date.

Grandmother avoids new-fangled remedies. What would she tell you about the following?

1 Water in which eggs have been boiled.

2 A cut in the hand between thumb and first finger.

3 Sleeping on the left side of the body.

4 The use for cobwebs.

5 A potato kept in the pocket.

6 Walking a sick child near a gasworks.

7 Mushrooms which will not blacken a silver spoon when cooking.

8 Drinking from the wrong side of the glass.

9 Rubbing a gold ring on the eye.

10 Inhaling the smell from a bad drain.

answers overleaf

1 'Causes warts' Witches used eggshells for boats when putting to sea. Warts have long been associated with witches, and the water in which eggs were boiled was soon believed to produce the warts themselves. This superstition persists and wart 'charming' is still carried out.

2 'Causes lockjaw' Lockjaw is caused by a germ called the tetanus bacillus. It lives in the intestines of animals and occurs in cultivated soils. It may enter any open wound of the body – regardless of site – and produce this disease..The hand has no special significance in lockjaw.

3 'Bad for the heart' The heart lies in the centre of the body. Its apex beats against the chest wall on the left and can be felt there. This gives rise to the mistaken belief that 'the heart is on the left side'. Sleeping on the left side is no more harmful to the heart than sleeping on the right.

4 'To stop bleeding' A wisp of cotton wool will stop bleeding from a cut and a cobweb can act in a similiar manner. On no account should cobwebs be used for this purpose. They are accumulations of dirt and are laden with germs. To place them on an open cut is highly dangerous.

5 'Prevents rheumatism' Faith can move mountains and undoubtedly keeps away odd aches and pains from those who walk around with potatoes in their pockets. Such aches and pains do not form a specific disease and are labelled 'rheumatism' by their owners for want of a better name.

6 'Cures whooping cough' The smell of a gasworks is often suggestive of disinfectant. From this, the idea quite wrongly arose that the odours had antiseptic properties, and if inhaled could cure whooping cough. Neither the smell from a gasworks nor the vapours from a tar machine have any curative function.

7 'Safe to eat' This test is no proof that a mushroom may be safely eaten. Like most kitchen tests for edibility, it is quite unreliable. Edible mushrooms must be expertly identified before taking them into a kitchen. If any doubt exists they should be thrown away.

8 'Cures hiccups' Hiccups are caused by involuntary contractions of the diaphragm – the flat sheet of muscle separating the chest from the abdomen. Air is suddenly forced through the voice box and produces the familiar sound. Drinking can sometimes help, but is quite independent of the side of the glass used.

9 'Cures a stye' A stye is a miniature abscess, usually formed at the base of an eyelash. Like abscesses elsewhere, the inflammation may on occasion disperse without discharging. More often, the stye bursts and evacuates its pus. The course in either instance is uninfluenced by the gold ring technique.

10 'Causes diphtheria' The smell from a bad drain is due to decomposing proteins and can be violently repugnant. Primitive fear sought in it the cause of the dreaded disease diphtheria. This disease is caused by a bacterium unrelated to the drain, and is nowadays rare due to immunization.

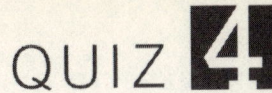
Brevity in medicine

'Words of learned length and thund'ring sound' are characteristic of any medical textbook. In practice, abbreviations save time and make life a lot easier. To ask for dichlorodiphenyltrichloroethane when needing a little DDT requires the dexterity of an acrobat and the patience of a saint.

Below are some fairly common medical abbreviations. Can you say what each one means?

1 MS

2 HIV

3 ECT

4 TB

5 GMC

6 CNS

7 GPI

8 FRCS

9 TPR

10 DT

answers overleaf

1 Multiple sclerosis This condition was far better known by its earlier name of disseminated sclerosis since the lesions of the nervous system are 'disseminated in time and space'. The illness is characterized by relapse and remission. The cause lies in a breakdown of the insulating fatty sheath of the nerve fibres.

2 Human immunodeficiency virus This virus is the forerunner of the disease AIDS (Acquired Immunodeficiency Syndrome). Infection by the virus may produce the typical symptoms of an acute fever or again may produce no symptoms at all. AIDS is liable to follow such viral infection after an interval of several years.

3 Electroconvulsive therapy This is the 'electric treatment' of psychiatry. It is of particular value in treating depressive states. Under anaesthesia, electrodes are placed on each temple, and a current is passed momentarily through the brain. About 15 minutes later, the patient wakes without recollection of the procedure.

4 Tuberculosis This disease was called 'consumption' by earlier generations. It is an infection by a microbe named the tubercle bacillus. It can attack many parts of the body but frequently settles in the lungs. Modern methods have proved particularly successful in preventing and curing tuberculosis. However, largely due to international travel, a serious resurgence of this disease is now making its presence known again in Britain.

5 General Medical Council This Council was established by Act of Parliament in 1858. It is responsible for keeping the official Medical Register and acts as a court of justice in medical matters. It is further required to supervise medical education and to prepare the *British Pharmacopoeia*.

6 Central nervous system The CNS consists of brain and spinal cord only. It does not include the other nerves. It is the central core of the nervous system and coordinates the body's function by receiving and despatching nervous impulses. It lies within the skull and vertebral column.

7 General paralysis of the insane This condition, so common in earlier times, is now fortunately rare. It is the result of syphilis of the brain. Striking changes in the patient's personality are liable to occur, often with grandiose delusions of great wealth and power. Ultimately, the disease produces complete paralysis and insanity.

8 Fellow of the Royal College of Surgeons On completing the examinations of this College, a specialist in surgery is granted a Fellowship and adds the letters FRCS to his name. By courtesy, he is addressed as Mr instead of Dr. This custom survives from days when surgeons were not medically qualified but were drawn from the ranks of barbers.

9 Temperature, pulse and respiration TPR charts are kept routinely in hospital wards and are recorded at intervals throughout the day. A patient's condition may be rapidly assessed from the information they give. The patterns of the recordings can be diagnostic of the illness. This is well seen in different kinds of malaria.

10 Delirium tremens This disease occurs in alcoholics, often after heavy drinking without food. Vivid visual hallucinations occur and may take the form of rats, bats, snakes or pink elephants according to individual taste. Marked trembling of the hands is present. Recovery usually follows in a few days. Occasionally, the condition proves fatal.

Seen at the circus

Human freaks found in circus side-shows can be of great medical interest. They represent well-known clinical conditions rarely seen in everyday life. In normal living, their disabilities would prove severe, yet the circus provides a special environment where many manage to lead successful lives.

    To what extent can you explain these well-known types of freak?

1 Tom Thumb

2 The India-rubber man

3 Siamese twins

4 The bearded lady

5 The sword swallower

6 The porcupine man

7 The fat lady

8 Broken glass and red hot cinder dancers

9 The giant

10 The wolf boy

answers overleaf

1 Pituitary undersecretion These people are pituitary dwarfs. They are alert, intelligent and well proportioned on a miniature scale. The pituitary gland at the base of the brain has failed to function normally during early years and has secreted too little of the growth hormone.

2 Lax joints This agile contortionist can place his limbs and body in fantastic positions. He has extreme laxity of the ligaments which bind his joints. Additional bony defects may be present. This condition may run in families and the grotesque range of movements be increased by practice from infancy.

3 Conjoined twins These twins arise by an incomplete separation of a single fertilized ovum. Two individuals then develop who at some point remain joined together. The possibility of surgical separation depends on the nature and site of this junction. The original twins, who were widely exhibited, were born in Siam in 1811.

4 Endocrine disturbance Bearded ladies have a disturbance of the endocrine system. The adrenal glands, sitting one on each kidney, are usually at fault. Overactivity by the outer portions of these glands produces masculinization of an adult woman. The beard is but one of several characteristic symptoms.

5 Reflex inhibition The sword swallower first learns to suppress the vomiting reflex when passing blunt objects into his throat. With further practice he manipulates them down his gullet and finally into his stomach. Eventually the skilled performer will dispose of approximately two feet of sword blade in this fashion.

6 Skin anomaly In this rare disease, ichthyosis sebacea spinosa, the lubricating glands of the skin are deficient. The body's surface from birth is dry, rough, cracked and scaly. The scales coalesce forming horny masses, and prolongation of these masses forms the spiny processes of the 'porcupine skin'.

7 Gross obesity Obesity has many causes which range from glands to gluttony. For side-show exhibition, the cause is unimportant but the effect must be maximal. Once up to weight, much food and no exercise would keep one in professional trim. Such overweight throws a severe strain on the body and paves the way to an early grave.

8 Hyperkeratosis of the feet Very thick skin on the soles of the feet enables these antics to be performed. By running barefoot under all conditions, the soles of the feet harden like leather. The skin acquires a horny layer which will protect the feet from the broken glass and permit rapid movement over glowing cinders.

9 Pituitary oversecretion The pituitary gland is again responsible – this time by oversecretion of the growth hormone during the growing years. Giants eight and nine feet tall can result. In spite of their impressive stature, these people are not robust and seldom live to any great age.

10 'Mowgli' fable Stories of infants fostered by wolves have a special appeal to popular superstition. Exhibitions of alleged 'wolf boys' occur from time to time. In spite of their spectacular representation, the claims of the showmen have never been substantiated by scientific enquiry.

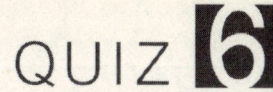

Fun with the flowers

The art of healing with herbs and plants has been known for centuries. Folklore developed it and witchcraft exploited it. Elegant accounts of its mysteries are found in the Herbals of the Middle Ages. From this art has evolved our modern science of pharmacology.

Many plants are still renowned for the drugs they contain. Which drugs would you associate with the following botanical specimens?

1 Oriental poppy

2 Henbane

3 Seaweed

4 Seeds of nux vomica

5 Coca shrub

6 Indian hemp

7 Californian buckthorn

8 Monkshood

9 Cinchona bark

10 Foxglove

answers overleaf

1 Opium Opium is the dried juice from the unripe seed capsules of the Oriental poppy *Papaver somniferum*. The ecstatic effects of smoking or eating its dark, resinous lumps have been known for thousands of years. Opium is a mixture of many powerful drugs, including the painkiller morphine.

2 Hyoscine This drug has a marked sedative action on the central nervous system and can be used to control maniacal behaviour. With morphine it will produce 'twilight sleep', and in combination with hydrobromide is effective against travel sickness. Concoctions of henbane were drunk at witches' Sabbaths.

3 Iodine Iodine is obtained from the ash of seaweed which has been dried and burnt. It has a wide range of uses in medicine. Dissolved in alcohol, it forms the disinfectant familiar to households for treating cuts and scratches. Iodine is employed for X-ray photography, and may be taken in disease of the thyroid gland.

4 Strychnine The large flat seeds of nux vomica contain strychnine, an important stimulant of the nervous system. It is a powerful poison, producing convulsions of the body and contortions of the face into a sardonic grin. It has a bitter taste and death can follow in a matter of minutes.

5 Cocaine Natives in the silver mines of the Andes found they could allay fatigue by chewing coca leaves. This is a secondary property of cocaine, well known as a local anaesthetic. It is a dangerous drug of addiction causing widely dilated pupils and sensations as if insects were crawling over the skin.

6 Marihuana This drug is also called hashish or cannabis. It is incorporated in certain paints for corns on the feet. When swallowed or smoked ('reefer' cigarettes) it produces a state of fatuous excitement followed by sleep with lurid dreams. The hemp plant is used in the manufacture of canvas and rope.

7 Cascara Cascara sagrada is Spanish and means 'sacred bark'. The bark comes from the Californian buckthorn and contains the drug. Cascara is a purgative, used in the treatment of constipation. It is usually prepared as a pill containing the dry extract of the bark.

8 Aconite Witches favoured this in their 'flying ointment', which was smeared on their bodies when attempting flight through the air. Monkshood is also known as wolfsbane, and its root resembles that of horseradish. Aconite is rarely used today except in dentistry. It was formerly given to promote sweating and reduce fever.

9 Quinine Cinchona bark originally came from Peru. It was introduced to Europe by Jesuit priests for the treatment of malaria. This 'Jesuits' bark' is the source of quinine, which is active against parasites found in the blood in attacks of malaria. Quinine reduces fever and, by its bitter flavour, can stimulate appetite.

10 Digitalis The leaves of the purple foxglove have long been employed by herbalists as a cure for 'dropsy' – that fluid which accumulates in the body when the heart is failing. These leaves contain the drug digitalis which strengthens the heart and increases its efficiency, allowing dispersal of the accumulated fluid.

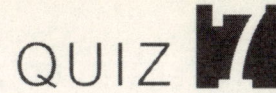

Praise famous men

Each person named here has made a great contribution to medical knowledge. In some cases, the discovery followed endless thought and careful experimentation. In others — no less great — it was made by pure chance. All have played a major part in the advancement of knowledge and its consequent relief of human suffering.

    Can you name those contributions for which these men are famous?

1 William Harvey (1578–1657)

2 Joseph Lister (1827–1912)

3 Andreas Vesalius (1514–1564)

4 James Simpson (1811–1870)

5 Edward Jenner (1749–1823)

6 Wilhelm Roentgen (1845–1923)

7 Alexander Fleming (1881–1955)

8 Patrick Manson (1844–1922)

9 Robert Koch (1843–1910)

10 Carl Gustav Jung (1875–1961)

answers overleaf

1 Circulation of the blood Harvey discovered the circulation of the blood. His experimental methods established a new approach for scientific enquiry. His findings on the heart and circulation were brilliantly set out in his book *De Motu Cordis*, published whilst Harvey was physician to Charles I.

2 Antisepsis Lister revolutionized surgery by his introduction of antisepsis. Hitherto, septic pus had been considered necessary and desirable in wound healing. Too often it had proved the precursor of death. Lister's technique dramatically reduced the death rate and made possible extensive operative surgery.

3 Human anatomy Vesalius demonstrated the true structure of the body. As Professor at Padua he challenged and corrected gross anatomical errors which had been accepted for centuries. He established the truth by human dissections and published his illustrated treatise *De Humani Corporis Fabrica* in 1543.

4 Anaesthesia James Simpson, Professor of Midwifery at Edinburgh, demonstrated anaesthesia by chloroform in 1847. Until this period, operations were terrifying experiences in which the screaming patient was tied down with ropes. With the advent of anaesthesia, a new era dawned for surgical treatment.

5 Vaccination Edward Jenner, a Gloucestershire practitioner, discovered vaccination. He observed that dairymaids who had had the mild disease of cowpox were spared the ravages of smallpox. Jenner began experimental inoculation with cowpox (vaccination). His efforts were completely successful and have led to the saving of countless lives.

6 X-rays Roentgen's discovery of X-rays in 1895 enabled bones in the body to be photographed and at once changed surgical methods and the diagnosis of fractures. Bones impede X-rays and cast the familiar shadows seen on the photographic film. Modern X-ray technique has extended widely and is now used for all parts of the body.

7 Penicillin Alexander Fleming discovered penicillin in 1928. A spore of the mould penicillium contaminated one of his bacterial culture plates. As the mould grew, surrounding colonies of dangerous bacteria were killed off. Treatment of patients with penicillin was made possible by Howard Florey's work at Oxford and followed in 1941.

8 Causes of malaria Manson demonstrated the role of the mosquito in producing the disease malaria. This disease had been thought – as its name implies – to result from the 'bad air' of ill-drained regions. These, of course, are the breeding ground of the mosquito. Eradication of this insect breaks the infection cycle and has freed large areas from the disease.

9 Tuberculosis germ Humanity owes a special debt to Robert Koch. Not only did this bacteriologist discover the germs of anthrax and cholera, but in 1882 identified the cause of tuberculosis. This long, slender organism is the tubercle bacillus – often known as Koch's bacillus. Koch's methods laid the foundations of modern bacteriology.

10 Analytical psychology The distinguished Swiss psychiatrist, Carl Gustav Jung, broke away from the school of psychoanalysis in 1912 to found his own school of analytical psychology. Much of Jung's theory concerns myths and mysticism. He gave us the concepts of 'complex' and 'collective unconscious' and to him we owe the words 'introvert' and 'extravert' in consideration of personality.

Fact and fiction

Truth may be stranger than fiction but sometimes the two are not easily distinguished. Tall stories, like rumours, increase with the telling and by repetition assume in time an air of authenticity.

These statements include both fact and fiction; but can you tell which is which?

1 Hair grows after death.

2 A fright during pregancy can produce a corresponding birthmark on the baby.

3 A hot iron and brown paper are good for lumbago.

4 Flowers must be removed from a bedroom at night.

5 A 'no salt' diet reduces weight.

6 Boils should be squeezed.

7 Burnt toast is good for diarrhoea.

8 A hot bath should not be taken immediately after a meal.

9 Stuff a cold and starve a fever.

10 Laugh and grow fat.

answers overleaf

1 Fiction Hair does not grow after death. Shrinkage and retraction of the skin may push the hair roots out a little, making them appear more conspicuous. Colourful legends of Napoleon and others growing beards in their tombs could well be explained by the potency of French wine!

2 Fiction A vivid imagination will read much in a baby's birthmark, just as inkblots or tea leaves can be read. Susceptible mothers are liable to accept the pronouncement made, and then obligingly think up some causative fright to fit the story. Frights cannot account for birthmarks in this superstitious fashion.

3 Fact Lumbago may be eased with heat of any kind. A hot iron is excellent – though an electric fire is equally useful. The brown paper can claim no magic properties. It is a necessary safety precaution when heating the iron has been left to the enthusiast.

4 Fiction Flowers breathe oxygen just like ourselves, but the amount is relatively small. Most draughty bedrooms have more than enough oxygen both for their sleepers and their flowers, even with all windows closed. No convincing case can be made to justify the ritual of putting the flowers outside.

5 Fact Table salt contains much sodium and tends to retain fluid within the body. Extra water means extra weight. When slimming or in certain diseases, salt intake may be reduced or cut out completely. Substitutes for flavouring food but which do not retain water can be obtained.

6 Fiction On no account should a boil be squeezed to accelerate its rupture, no matter how gratifying this procedure may appear. In so doing, infection is forced under pressure into healthy tissues. Boils on the nose or upper lip are particularly dangerous. Squeezing here may give rise to a fatal brain thrombosis.

7 Fact Burnt toast forms charcoal. Charcoal is particularly effective in absorbing poisons from the digestive tract and will assist diarrhoea arising from this cause. This fact has been of considerable help to explorers and travellers when normal medical aid has been unobtainable.

8 Fact After a meal, as much blood as is able circulates to the gut to assist digestion. In a hot bath, blood flows to the body's surface for cooling purposes. A combined demand by both processes is liable to leave insufficient blood to circulate to the brain. Dizziness and fainting may follow.

9 Fiction In fever, the appetite is poor but an adequate nutritional intake must be maintained. Fluids are of great importance, to replace those lost by sweating. 'Stuffing' has little effect on colds which improve in their own time anyway. Many colds are of course mild fevers.

10 Fiction No one can explain exactly what laughter is and there is no evidence that it makes one grow fat. It is an excellent tonic and dispels tension and apprehension. Worry and stress may cause obesity through compulsive overeating. On this basis, laugh and grow slim. Stout people may have a constitutional tendency towards jolliness.

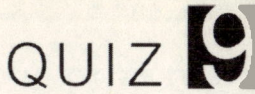

Brains' trust

Brains have come much into fashion nowadays. Educationalists assess them, psychiatrists unveil them, electronic engineers construct them and politicians wash them. But for all their efforts, our detailed knowledge of this incredible organ still remains severely limited.

How far does your own knowledge enable you to answer these ten questions on the brain?

1 Is fish specially good for the brain?

2 What is 'grey matter'?

3 Are our brains hollow?

4 Are male brains heavier then female?

5 Can 'brain waves' be recorded?

6 What is a 'brain storm'?

7 Why are the surfaces of our brains corrugated?

8 Does a high forehead indicate intelligence?

9 What is 'water on the brain'?

10 What is 'softening of the brain'?

answers overleaf

1 No The brain derives no special advantage from a fish diet. No-one would deny that fish is an excellent food that is rich in protein. The liver oils contain vitamins A and D, and fish roes are highly nutrient. These benefits are available to the whole body. To link fish with an idea of increased brain activity is quite wrong.

2 Cerebral cortex Grey matter is the cerebral cortex. This is found at the surface of the brain and consists of millions of nerve cells packed in layers. The cortex is related to consciousness. Our higher faculties are dependent on the healthy function of the grey matter.

3 Yes Our brains are hollowed by a system of cavities lying deep within their substance. These cavities are the ventricles of the brain and are four in number. Leonardo da Vinci demonstrated the ventricles by injections of wax.

4 Yes Male brains weigh more than female but, gratifying though this might first appear, greater weight does not imply superior function. The brain of an adult weighs approximately 3 lbs. Many of the world's finest brains have weighed less than average.

5 Yes Brain activity is accompanied by miniature electrical changes. A sensitive instrument is employed to record these from the scalp and to reproduce them as a wave-tracing known as the electroencephalogram. In health, the brain waves show recognized patterns. In brain disease, their changes can be diagnostic.

6 Non-specific term This vague term has no precise medical meaning. It is used in everyday life to indicate any state of mental confusion which occurs with sudden onset. Such confusional episodes have a wide variety of causes which range from psychological stress to organic disease of the brain.

7 Increase of surface area The corrugations of the brain enormously increase its surface area and, therefore, the amount of grey matter. Millions of extra brain cells are thereby accommodated and produce a corresponding superior performance. In this lies a great difference between human and animal brains. Many animal brains have quite smooth surfaces.

8 No High foreheads do not indicate intelligence. Their shape is determined by bone and not by the brain. The appearance of a high forehead may be more impressive, but for performance it can claim no special advantage over a low brow. A receding hairline often accentuates the shape of the forehead.

9 Hydrocephalus This is an excessive accumulation of cerebrospinal fluid within the skull. The increase in pressure may be very great, forcing apart the cranial bones of a young child and causing considerable enlargement of the head. The brain tissue may be damaged by compression and mental deficiency is liable to follow.

10 Cerebral degeneration Old age, disease or damage to the brain may cause death of its nerve cells in certain areas. As the cells die, they liquify and are later replaced by a form of scar tissue. This liquifying process is 'softening of the brain'. It is frequently accompanied by mental deterioration.

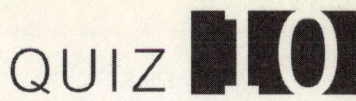
Rock-a-bye baby

A baby's birth is the best excuse for a celebration. Months of speculation have suddenly ended. Boy or girl? Where and when? One or several? Who — sometimes what — is it going to look like? Well, the suspense is over and at least one knows the worst.

The next generation is already on the way. Just how well informed are you in this remarkable process?

1 What is a 'breech delivery'?

2 What is 'witch's milk'?

3 A baby is sometimes born with 'a hole in the heart'. What is this condition?

4 What is a 'phantom pregnancy'?

5 What is a 'Caesarean birth'?

6 How do twins arise?

7 What is a 'caul'?

8 Which common infection can be critical for a mother in early pregnancy?

9 What is the rhesus factor?

10 What is the Ascheim–Zondek reaction?

answers overleaf

1 Arrival upside-down Babies are conservative of habit and in most cases are born head first. Occasionally, the individualist presents upside-down and, in spite of discouragement, persists in this attitude. Birth with the buttocks leading is termed a 'breech'. Delivery in skilled hands proceeds quite normally.

2 Infant 'lactation' A mother in labour has hormones in her blood which prepare her for lactation and feeding her child. These sometimes react on the breast tissue of the infant, producing a transient discharge from the baby's nipples. Such secretion from the breast of the newly born is called 'witch's milk'.

3 Cardiac septal defect In a healthy human heart the right side is partitioned completely from the left. The dividing septum ensures that blood in the two sides cannot mix. Occasionally, a child is born with a defect in this partition — the so-called 'hole in the heart'. The condition is critical and requires advanced cardiac surgery.

4 Pseudocyesis On occasion, a woman wishing desperately to bear a child may feel certain she is pregnant when this is not the case. Her conviction may be so great that certain physical changes occur, which closely simulate the signs of pregnancy. Queen Mary I was a famous example. The condition is known as pseudocyesis or 'phantom pregnancy'.

5 Birth by operation Delivery is obtained by lifting the infant through an incision in the mother's abdominal wall. The child is spared the passage through its mother's bony pelvis. Although this practice has been known since earliest times, the allegation that Julius Caesar was born in this way is without foundation.

6 Anomalous fertilization Identical twins are formed by the splitting of one fertilized ovum to form two individuals. Such twins are alike in every way. Twins may also form by the individual fertilization of two separate ova. Such twins are not identical and bear the same relationship to each other as normal brothers and sisters.

7 Retained membranes on the infant's head A portion of the birth membranes may sometimes be retained on the infant's head as it is born. This is the caul and is believed by the superstitious to be very lucky. In particular, it is considered to protect against drowning and has often been in demand with sailors. Dickens' David Copperfield was born with a caul.

8 German measles A pregnant woman must be protected from risk of infection with German measles. The virus causing this disease is known to affect the formation of the child within the womb. For this reason, an infection with German measles during the first three months of pregnancy is considered grave.

9 Blood agglutinogen This is an agglutinogen factor found in human blood. Those who possess it are called rhesus positive the few who do not are rhesus negative. Its clinical importance lies in blood transfusion and obstetrics. Special care and precautions must be taken with a rhesus-negative woman pregnant with a rhesus-positive child.

10 Pregnancy test Certain hormones are released into an expectant mother's blood and ultimately pass into her urine. If this urine is injected into immature female mice, striking and characteristic changes occur. This phenomenon was therefore used as a test for early pregnancy. It is known as the Ascheim–Zondek reaction.

QUIZ

Queen Anne's dead

Most people know that Queen Anne's dead, but very few know just how she died. Death is important to medicine; its study, paradoxically enough, has prolonged life and has aided the unending quest for the elimination of disease.

Each of these well-known persons met an unusual and sudden death. But can you say how?

1 Socrates

2 Sir Roger Casement

3 Joan of Arc

4 Hermann Goering

5 Cleopatra

6 Percy Bysshe Shelley

7 Marie Antoinette

8 Julius Caesar

9 Abraham Lincoln

10 King John

answers overleaf

1 Hemlock poisoning Socrates, the Greek philosopher, was condemned to death. In prison, he drank the traditional 'cup of hemlock'. Hemlock poisoning produces an ascending muscular paralysis. This starts in the legs and creeps slowly up the body until breathing is no longer possible. The mind remains surprisingly clear throughout.

2 Judicial hanging This form of capital punishment is designed for instantaneous death. A physical assessment is made of the individual, and the mechanics of the execution are carefully calculated. Judicial hanging results in a fracture or dislocation of the upper cervical vertebrae. The spinal cord is destroyed close to its junction with the vital centres of the brain.

3 Burnt at the stake Joan of Arc was burnt at Rouen in 1431. This inhuman form of execution was favoured for heretics. Undoubtedly, most succumbed to the fumes before the flames actually reached them. Shock, asphyxia and carbon monoxide poisoning would account for the majority of deaths by burning.

4 Cyanide poisoning Potassium cyanide is a deadly poison derived from Prussic acid. Its action upon the cells of the body destroys their vital processes and leaves them incapable of utilizing the oxygen of the blood. This action is immediate and symptoms can appear within seconds. The smell of bitter almonds is characteristic of this poisoning.

5 Snakebite Cleopatra, according to legend, died from the bite of an asp. The body's tissues absorb snake venom with great rapidity and disastrous consequences are liable to follow. These may include internal bleeding or paralysis of the nervous system. Antivenoms are now available and should be used for snakebites whenever possible.

6 Drowning Shelley was drowned in the Italian Gulf of Spezia in 1822. Death from drowning is most commonly caused by asphyxia. Air cannot enter the lungs and respiration is impossible. On rare occasions, death can be instantaneous; it follows reflexly from the impact of water on the larynx or nasal spaces.

7 Guillotined This Queen of France died on the guillotine at Paris in 1793. Decapitation by such execution had been proposed generally for France some years earlier by Dr Guillotin, a French physician. Although the machine bears his name, Dr Guillotin did not invent it nor, as is often thought, did he die on it.

8 Multiple stab wounds Caesar was murdered in the Senate House at Rome on the Ides of March in 44 BC. His attackers' swords caused numerous haemorrhages and his wounds were found principally in the chest, abdomen and back. Some undoubtedly penetrated vital organs. Unconsciousness would occur rapidly from loss of blood. Death would follow shortly after.

9 Shot Abraham Lincoln was shot at close quarters whilst in a box at the theatre. Examination of such gunshot wounds reveals much to an experienced eye. The sites of the bullet's entry and exit each bear distinct and characteristic features. These can indicate the type of firearm used, the direction from which fired and the approximate range.

10 Surfeit of lampreys Having lost his crown jewels in the Wash, King John was greatly peeved. Like many another, he sought solace in the comfort mechanism of eating. He had peaches, which some say were poisoned, and combined these with too many lampreys, which proved his undoing. One can never be too careful of seafood!

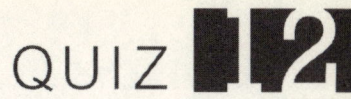

Ailment-itis

Medicine, as everyone knows, makes much use of the suffix *itis*. This forms a quick and convenient way of denoting inflammation – the body's fundamental reaction to injury of any kind.

Everyone knows that an inflamed appendix is 'appendicitis'. But what is the condition called when inflammation occurs in the...?

1 Skin

2 Liver

3 Stomach

4 Intestines

5 Bladder

6 Muscle sheaths

7 Brain

8 Vein

9 Nerves

10 Tongue

answers overleaf

1 Dermatitis Housewives who wash up in strong detergents may easily develop this condition. Grease is removed from the plates and natural oils from the skin. Hands and arms become roughened, cracked and painful. Industry protects its workers from harmful chemicals, many of which would produce severe dermatitis.

2 Hepatitis Inflammation of the liver occurs in illnesses of widely different origin. Virus infections, phosphorous poisoning and malaria are some examples. A chronic hepatitis occurs in alcoholics and many of the liver cells die. They are replaced by fibrous tissue which may give rise to the condition of cirrhosis or 'hobnail liver'.

3 Gastritis Inflammation of the stomach often occurs when we have eaten something which has 'disagreed' with us. The effects of unripe apples and alcoholic excesses are everyday knowledge. Until the condition clears, the stomach remains abnormally sensitive, irritable, and shows difficulty in digesting its food.

4 Enteritis Many tropical diseases can produce a severe enteritis, with diarrhoea a leading symptom. Cholera, dysentery and typhoid are classical examples. Fluid is passed from the body to the bowel in excessive quantities. Unless adequate replacements of fluid are drunk, the body becomes rapidly dehydrated.

5 Cystitis More common in women than in men, this condition frequently follows an infection. Sometimes the bladder develops small pockets in its walls where bacteria congregate in stagnant urine. Recurrent attacks of cystitis may occur during pregnancy but the condition clears after the birth of the child.

6 Fibrositis This form of 'muscular rheumatism' can strike with lightning-like rapidity and is very common in Britain. A stiff neck and lumbago are variations of the condition. Surprisingly, little is really known about this disease or the reason for its very sudden onset. Quickest relief is found in the application of heat.

7 Encephalitis Inflammation of the brain gives cause for grave concern. Its early symptoms of fever, headache and vomiting can be followed by coma and death. Residual brain damage may still be found when the acute stages have passed. The cause is most commonly a viral infection and may originate from such everyday diseases as measles, mumps and chickenpox.

8 Phlebitis Inflamed veins are complicated by the clotting of blood which occurs within them. This situation may have serious consequences and is one which requires careful attention. Phlebitis is liable to be found in varicose veins. The vein is usually painful and tender and may sometimes be felt as a thickened cord.

9 Neuritis Neuritic symptoms vary considerably according to the anatomical nerve affected. Feelings of numbness, tingling and diminshed sensation are often combined with some loss of muscle power. The condition may follow injury, infection, poisoning or vitamin deficiency. Chronic alcoholics are particularly prone to neuritis.

10 Glossitis A temporary glossitis will follow a 'burnt tongue', when food or drink has been taken too hot for the mouth. More persistent glossitis may occur as a sign of pernicious anaemia or certain other anaemic states. The tongue becomes smooth, shiny and may be sore. A very similiar picture is found in deficiency of vitamin B.

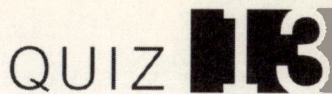

Answer anatomically

Oddities abound within the fabric of the human body. Such is the stuff of which we are made. Though some are visible from the body's surface, most are revealed only by dissection.

Here are listed ten quaint features of the human body. Can you say what these really are?

1 Adam's apple

2 Cockles of the heart

3 Solar plexus

4 Anatomical snuffbox

5 Hamstrings

6 Turkish saddle

7 Funny bone

8 Floating ribs

9 Gooseflesh

10 Alderman's nerve

answers overleaf

1 Laryngeal prominence The Adam's apple forms a familiar surface landmark on the front of the throat, more obvious in men than in women. It is a prominence of the larynx, the organ responsible for voice production and which houses the vocal cords. On swallowing, the larynx moves freely and the excursions of the 'apple' are easily seen.

2 Valves of the heart The valves of the heart and its great vessels bear a resemblance to cockle shells, and for years were assigned a mystic significance. Their construction permits the flow of blood in one direction only. Entering from the great veins, blood passes through the chambers of the heart and is expelled at high pressure into the arteries.

3 Abdominal nerve centre The solar plexus is a large nerve centre found in the abdomen. It lies between the kidneys on one of the principle arteries. Its name is derived from the appearance of its nerve fibres which radiate outwards like rays from the sun. These fibres are distributed to the abdominal organs.

4 At the side of the wrist A pit can be felt where the creases of the wrist wind round and cross the two main tendons to the back of the thumb. It is most obvious when the thumb is forcibly extended backwards. Its convenience in holding snuff before sniffing has given it the name of the 'anatomical snuffbox'.

5 Tendons of the knee The hamstrings are the prominent tendons felt at the back of the knee on each side just above the joint. They are attached to important muscles of the back of the thigh and are responsible for flexing the knee. 'Hamstringing' by cutting these tendons would render the legs quite useless.

6 In the skull floor The 'sella turcica' or Turkish saddle is a part of the sphenoid bone found in the base of the skull. It resembles a miniature saddle with pommel, seat and cantle. In it sits the pituitary gland – the master gland of internal secretion – which is attached to the base of the brain.

7 Medial epicondyle of humerus The so-called 'funny bone' is a projection from the inner side of the elbow, technically known as the medial epicondyle of the humerus. This projection is not unduly sensitive but winding round it, in an exposed position, is the ulnar nerve. A blow here numbs the nerve and produces the drastic subjective sensations.

8 Eleventh and twelfth ribs Twelve ribs are situated on each side of the body. They articulate behind with the vertebral column. In front, the upper ten ribs are firmly secured either to the breast bone or to an adjacent rib. In contrast, the lowest two on each side are quite free anteriorly. For this reason they are known as the floating ribs.

9 Cutaneous muscular contraction Goose flesh is produced by a mass contraction of countless tiny muscles which lie within the skin. Each is attached to the root of a hair. These muscles respond involuntarily to cold or fright. Goose flesh is the vestigial human counterpart of the erection of fur or ruffling of feathers frequently observed in animals.

10 Auricular branch of the vagus nerve The tenth cranial nerve is the vagus, meaning 'wanderer'. It supplies the stomach but sends a small special branch which innervates the ear – the Alderman's nerve. These good trenchermen when replete at banquet dropped a little cold water into their ears. By reflex action, stomach movements increased and made room for further onslaught on subsequent courses.

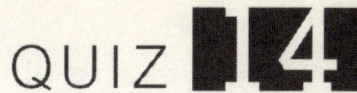
Tongue twisters

This selection of words will twist your tongue. Among them are some of the most formidable found in medical terminology. Can you suggest what any of these mean? In some cases, the answers are disarmingly simple. Don't be discouraged if your score is low. It is hoped they will add to your medical knowledge – if not to your everyday vocabulary!

1 Amnesia

2 Phthisis

3 Dysdiadochokinesis

4 Achromatopsia

5 Onychogryphosis

6 Thyrotoxicosis

7 Rhinophyma

8 Cheiropompholyx

9 Achondroplasia

10 Bronchiectasis

answers overleaf

1 Memory loss Amnesia has many causes and these vary widely. Head injuries are commonly accompanied by memory loss for a period preceding the accident. In old age, recent events may be forgotten yet detailed accounts be given of the past. In different circumstances, Freud suggested we forget those things we are unwilling to remember.

2 Pulmonary tuberculosis In recent years, medical progress has revolutionized our attitude towards this illness. What was previously a death sentence now has every hope of cure. Protective inoculation has become possible. Mass miniature X-rays have favoured an early diagnosis and enabled treatment with streptomycin and its allied drugs to be started without delay.

3 Muscular incoordination Dysdiadochokinesis is an inability to make small repetitive movements very quickly – as for example rapid pronation and supination of the wrists or tapping the fingers very quickly upon a table. It is indicative of suspected disease of the cerebellum – the small brain which coordinates muscle movement.

4 Total colour blindness Complete absence of colour vision is very rare. When it occurs, the world is seen in shades of grey – rather like a black and white cinematograph film. Partial degrees of colour blindness are much more frequent. They occur predominantly in men and are usually found as a visual defect for red and green.

5 Griffin nail Occasionally, the growth of a nail on a finger or toe gets grossly out of control. It thickens enormously, darkens in colour and becomes excessively hard. Cutting by normal measures is quite impossible and the free edge of the nail may turn down like a claw. This is known as griffin nail or onychogryphosis.

6 Thyroid poisoning Like some furnace burning at full draught, hyperactivity of the thyroid gland can give rise to an intense acceleration of the body's processes. The heart races, the hands tremble and the body perspires. The eyes may stare wildly from the head. This condition responds well to treatment and the outlook, fortunately, is good.

7 'Bottle nose' Most of us have seen an unfortunate person with a marked overgrowth of the lower part of the nose. The condition is unmistakable and forms a conspicuous, lobulated mass in which the glands of the skin show prominently. The names 'bottle nose' and 'grog blossom' are ill-chosen and inappropriate. Contrary to popular ignorance, the condition is unrelated to drinking.

8 Blisters of the hands In the world of dermatology, cheiropompholyx denotes an eruption of blisters which breaks out on both hands. Its cause is not fully understood but is related to overactivity by the sweat glands. Such overactivity can have an underlying psychological cause. Similar eruptions are occasionally found on the feet.

9 Maldevelopment of bone Achondroplasia runs in certain families and is a failure of natural bone development. Those afflicted present a dwarf-like appearance. The bones of the limbs suffer most deformity and are severely stunted in growth. The face and head are usually spared and patients are in full possession of their mental faculties.

10 Bronchial dilatation The cause of this chronic chest condition is usually to be found in an earlier unresolved pneumonia. Degeneration occurs in the bronchi and bronchioles of the lung which dilate and act as pockets of infection. Coughing is persistent and breathing becomes difficult. The tips of the fingers take on a characteristic swelling known as 'clubbing' and give the fingers an appearance of stunted drumsticks.

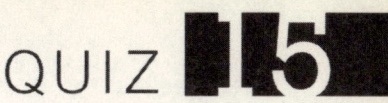
Down with everything!

Some people are never satisfied – nothing's right and everything's wrong. Most of us know how to put the world to rights with a few well-chosen words from a deep armchair. Grumbling, if properly done, is an accomplished art. All of us are anti-something but this quiz is anti-everything.

Each answer begins with the prefix *anti*. Supply the complete word in these cases.

1 Pencillin – the founder member of this group.

2 Sb

3 The basis of our immune system.

4 These stop the clot...

5 ...and these cool the hot!

6 The answer to allergy?

7 Grandma's poultice.

8 To prevent fits.

9 They thwart the poisoner.

10 Death to germs!

31

answers overleaf

1 Antibiotics Antibiotics are substances produced by fungi or bacteria which inhibit or destroy the life of other germs. Their discovery and use in medicine marked a major triumph in the fight against disease. Many diseases, hitherto fatal, have been rendered harmless by antibiotic therapy.

2 Antimony Sb is the chemical symbol for antimony, a metal closely related to arsenic. The ancients used it as a beauty preparation; later it became a fashionable poison. In the sixteenth century, a craze for prescribing antimony led to its widespread abuse and disrepute. Nowadays, it is used in the treatment of tropical diseases.

3 Antibodies These are modified blood proteins which are formed in response to stimulation by antigens. Many antigens are potentially harmful substances such as bacterial toxins and foreign proteins. The antibody is the counter-agent produced by the body which neutralizes or renders harmless the antigen. This is the fundamental reaction from which a state of immunity is built up.

4 Anticoagulants The untimely clotting of blood presents a grave problem in medicine. When occurring in the heart or brain, it may lead to sudden death. However, it has become possible to administer drugs which will suppress or delay the clotting process. These are the anticoagulants. Their use has saved the lives of many patients.

5 Antipyretics Antipyretics are drugs which reduce fever and bring down the body's temperature. They may do this by the promotion of sweating or by acting centrally upon the brain. The antipryretic aspirin is found in almost every home. Quinine, phenacetin and ipecacuanha are other members of this group.

6 Antihistamines In allergic disorders, a chemical substance called histamine is released by the tissues. Unpleasant symptoms rapidly follow. These may include a puffed-up face, streaming eyes, itching of the skin and nettlerash. The antihistamine drugs counter these effects and bring great relief. If taken prophylactically, they can forestall the occurrence of an allergic attack.

7 Antipholgistine This well-known proprietary paste makes an excellent poultice. It retains its heat for some hours after application and can bring speedy relief to deep-seated pain in the muscles, joints or tendons. It is composed largely of kaolin, to which a mixture of aromatic oils has been added.

8 Anticonvulsants These drugs have received much recent interest. They are used in the control of fits. Such fits are usually – but not invariably – of an epileptic kind. Phenobarbitone, phenytoin sodium and troxidone are anticonvulsants which have proved their effectiveness. Their success has stimulated much new activity in the treatment of epileptic disorders.

9 Antidotes Long lists of these medicinal counter-poisons are found in the textbooks of reference. Rarely is the book or the antidote at hand in the moment of crisis. The immediate treatment of poisoning is best conducted on general lines. Most lives are saved by inducing vomiting, washing out the stomach and sending at once for the doctor.

10 Antiseptics Antiseptics destroy germs. Their use is limited since the strong ones also destroy human tissues. Whenever possible, we now aim one better by using the technique of asepsis. This requires the rigid exclusion of germs by strict sterile precautions. Asepsis is vital for surgical work and has largely replaced the need for antiseptics.

Sense and nonsense

Nonsense, in the right place, can add great gaiety to life – as devotees of W. S. Gilbert are well aware. Nonsense, in the wrong place, is positively dangerous and this is never more true than in the field of medical knowledge.

Here is a mixture of sense and nonsense – can you sort out which is which?

1 Red flannel has special medicinal properties.

2 An apple a day keeps the doctor away.

3 Blood whipped with twigs will not clot.

4 Pinpricks are more dangerous than needle-pricks.

5 Aspirins induce sleep.

6 Our eyes view everything upside down.

7 A good price can be obtained for one's body by leaving it for dissection after death.

8 The brain is affected by the phases of the moon.

9 The smallest print is best read by short-sighted people.

10 Intelligence favours a frail physique.

answers overleaf

1 Nonsense Red, the colour of fire and blood, symbolizes life. Mediaeval cures frequently invoked red drapes and wrappings for the patient. The colour survives in medical university robes. Red flannel can claim no specific medicinal factor. Chilling of the body's surface can be prevented by any good quality flannel.

2 Nonsense Fresh fruit is an excellent source of vitamins, to which apples are no exception. In themselves, they possess no special properties for warding off the doctor; their ingestion at the unripe stage may demand the attention of a physician all too soon. Apples contain a high percentage of water. Their cellulose 'roughage' can greatly assist the normal function of the bowel.

3 Sense When freshly drawn blood is whipped with twigs, fibrin is rapidly deposited upon them. This protein exists in the circulating blood as fibrinogen. Its deposition on the twigs removes an essential factor of the clotting mechanism, and the defibrinated blood remains fluid.

4 Nonsense The risk is really equal. The danger lies not with the pin or needle but with the introduction of germs into the tissues. Germs are always present on the surface of the skin and will be found on any unsterile article. With sterile precautions, a prick from either pin or needle can be completely harmless.

5 Nonsense Contrary to popular belief, aspirins do not induce sleep. By the process of suggestion, faith in their ability to do so might well be enough to ensure a good night – but the same could be said for a bread pill. If sleeplessness is caused by pain, aspirin may be of great help. By relieving the pain, natural sleep can follow unimpeded.

6 Sense The lens of the eye is biconvex and will therefore throw a real, inverted image onto the retina. The world within our eye has turned completely upside down. Fortunately, the brain allows for this. A mental process re-inverts the picture and, without our realizing it, the status quo is miraculously restored.

7 Nonsense Bodies are not purchased in this manner. Hair-raising stories of rare diseases which increase the market value of a corpse are quite untrue. Traffic in the dead was stamped out after the murderous outrages of the early nineteenth century. Anyone wishing to leave their body to a medical school may do so. Dissection occurs in the course of routine anatomical instruction.

8 Nonsense A long-standing superstition affirms that the functioning of the brain can be adversely affected by the varying phases of the moon. The word 'lunatic' is derived from the Latin 'luna' meaning moon. There is no doubt that mental illness often shows phasic variations. To relate these to lunar influence is quite unjustifiable.

9 Sense Normal sight has its nearest point for clear vision approximately 25 centimetres from the eye. Short-sighted people can focus clearly on objects held much closer than this. The closer an object is to the eye, the larger the image formed on the retina. Thus, short-sighted persons can read tiny print inaccessible to the normal-sighted.

10 Nonsense Intelligence favours both the robust and frail. The sedentary scholar, who pores over books in an ill-ventilated library, may not present the same healthy appearance as a weather-beaten outdoor worker – but their intelligence may well be equal. By temperament, thin, frail-looking types (ectomorphs) often have a greater tendency to contemplative thinking.

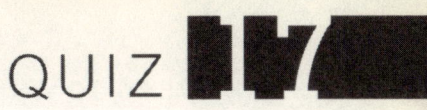

To catch you napping

The phenomenon of sleep is a fascinating one. Normally, we spend one-third of our lives in it. Its variance in sickness and in health can be remarkable. Just how or why we sleep are still unanswered questions. Theories abound and facts are many but definitive explanation remains as elusive as ever.

Sleep is the subject of this quiz. Assuming you are still awake, how many of these questions can you answer?

1 What is 'twilight sleep'?

2 What is sleeping sickness?

3 What is sleep treatment?

4 Who was the God of dreams?

5 Who wrote *The Interpretation of Dreams*?

6 What is sleepy sickness?

7 What is sleepwalking?

8 What are sleeping drugs?

9 What is 'sleepy dust'?

10 What is 'beauty sleep'?

answers overleaf

1 Analgesia for childbirth Obstetricians have used a combination of morphine with hyoscine to produce the state of 'twilight sleep' whilst the baby is born. Its action is twofold. Pain is diminished and memory is modified so that afterwards no recollection of pain remains. Though advantageous to the mother, this analgesia is not entirely without risk to the child.

2 Trypanosomiasis This dreaded disease of Africa is caused by microscopic blood parasites known as trypanosomes. These parasites are transmitted from the sick to the healthy by the bite of the blood-sucking tsetse fly. Infection spreads from the blood to the brain and gives rise to symptoms of increasing sleepiness which end in death.

3 Prolonged narcosis States of mental agitation and acute anxiety can benefit greatly from this therapy. Aided by hypnotics, the patient sleeps for as much as 20 hours each day for a period of days or even weeks. Meals and toilet requirements are dealt with during waking intervals. Mind and body are rested from the stress generated by the factors of the illness.

4 Morpheus This ancient god promoted sleep and was the creator of dreams. The drug morphine is named after him from the painless, carefree sleep associated with its action. Morphine is the chief alkaloid of opium. When taken, the pupil of the eye constricts to a pin-point. Its effect on mice causes their tails to stand straight up in the air.

5 Sigmund Freud Professor Freud's world-famous theory of dreams was published in 1900. He considered the dream, as we remember it, to be really a heavily disguised version of the true or 'latent' dream. This latter is produced by the unconscious mind and incorporates a wish fulfilment. The disguise is achieved by recognized mental mechanisms, including the free use of symbols.

6 Encephalitis lethargica Sleepy sickness is quite unrelated to African sleeping sickness mentioned above. These two diseases should not be confused. Sleepy sickness is encephalitis lethargica, a viral disease of the nervous system. Inflammation of the brain occurs with symptoms of increasing drowsiness. A serious epidemic swept Europe during World War I.

7 Somnambulism Many children sleepwalk at some time or other. Causes range widely from emotional upsets to digestive troubles. In most cases, this activity is a phase in normal development. With adults, sleepwalking is rarer and usually of psychological significance. A relationship exists between sleepwalking and hysteria.

8 Hypnotics Sleeping drugs depress the activity of the central nervous system, assisting the natural process of sleep. The barbiturate group of drugs was widely used for this purpose. Hypnotics of brief duration are of value to those who find difficulty in actually getting to sleep. Those of prolonged action ensure continuous sedation throughout the night. The benzodiazepine group now furnishes many modern hypnotics.

9 Conjunctival debris The deposits found in the corners of one's eye on waking are products of the eye's self-cleansing mechanism. During sleep, tears flow gently across the eye washing its surface and removing conjunctival debris. This mechanism explains the ease with which elusive foreign bodies in the eye become dislodged and removed during hours of sleep.

10 Sleep before midnight This sleep, we are told, does us the most good. When late nights play havoc with our looks, some early retiring does much to repair the damage. Can these hours before midnight claim special values of their own? The first hours of sleep are the deepest, but most benefit undoubtedly comes from the longer night's rest obtained.

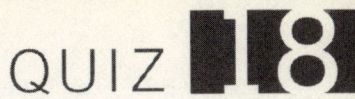
Apothecaries' cypher

Few people have not at some time or another been intrigued by the symbols and hieroglyphics of a prescription. The coded message is borne from doctor to pharmacist and, after translation, the medicine materializes. Today, having become metric, the older romance of prescribing has disappeared. These symbols and abbreviations belong to a past age and are now largely an anachronism.

Here are ten which were in common use. How many of them can you decypher?

1 ℨ

2 s.o.s.

3 Ʒ

4 a.c.

5 ʒ

6 m. ft. m.

7 ℳ

8 h.d.

9 ◯

10 B.P.

answers overleaf

1 A drachm Drachms may be solid or liquid. In Apothecaries' Weight, a drachm equals 60 grains and is, therefore, equivalent to one-eighth of an ounce. The term has an interesting history. Derived from Greek it was literally as much as could be grasped by the hand. A liquid drachm similarly equals one-eighth of a fluid ounce.

2 Si opus sit S.O.S. is not, as might be thought, an exhortation in the prescription for the saving of souls! It merely indicates that the medicine – such as for example a tranquilizer – should be taken 'should the occasion arise'!

3 A scruple Most curiously, a scruple was originally a sort of small pebble as might be found between the sandal and the foot – hence a difficulty obstructing action. It was probably used in counting and in Apothecaries' Weight one scruple was one-third of a drachm or the twenty-fourth part of an ounce.

4 Ante cibos This denotes that the medicine should be taken 'before food'. With certain medicines which are to be absorbed via the stomach wall, the process is obviously quicker and more effective if not impeded by the presence of food.

5 An ounce This term is derived from the Latin 'uncia' meaning a twelfth part and in Apothecaries' Weight, 12 ounces equal one pound. One ounce equals eight drachms, or 24 scruples. Similarly, a fluid ounce equals eight fluid drachms or 480 minims.

6 Misce fiat mistura This direction is 'to mix and make a mixture'. It would be found at the bottom of prescriptions where a number of ingredients had been specified. One famous prescription set out ingredients which when mixed would produce a Devil!

7 A minim In measurements of fluid, one minim corresponds to one drop. Sixty minims equal one fluid drachm and 480 minims equal one fluid ounce. In measurements of weight, a minim is equal to one grain.

8 Hora decubitus This means 'on going to bed'. It is a most important time for any attempts at healing. The different types of medicine taken on retiring to bed are legion but have the common task of effectively promoting the blessing of a sound and restorative night's sleep.

9 Octarius This signifies a fluid pint. It would appear to be of High Dutch origin signifying a measure of wine. It is the equivalent of 16 fluid ounces.

10 Brittanica Pharmacopoeia The *Brittanica Pharmacopoeia* is the exhaustive reference work which forms the 'bible' of pharmacy. Authorized by the Government, it constitutes the expert listing and setting of standards for all medications and their dosages.

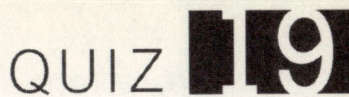
Rainbow wrangles

One of Nature's great gifts to mankind is our ability to appreciate colour. Its effect can greatly influence mood, feeling and even confidence – a phenomenon known as chromaesthesia.

Each answer to these clues contains a colour. We may not know where the rainbow ends but it begins right here at the first question.

1 A conservative infant.

2 Scourge of the fourteenth century.

3 But little boys get this too!

4 Communicated by a jaundiced Jack.

5 That dark drink!

6 Cosmetic for Lady Jane?

7 In aristocratic vein.

8 The kiddies' break?

9 The opposite to the man who won't strike with his workmates.

10 For a Royal see?

39

answers overleaf

1 Blue baby A baby is blue if its blood is inadequately oxygenated. In most of the sensational cases, a congenital deficiency of the heart or its vessels is present. Inefficient circulation through the lungs starves the blood of oxygen and it darkens in colour. Fully oxygenated blood is bright red.

2 Black death Of all plagues in the history of mankind, this was the worst. It devastated Europe in the fourteenth century, killing millions of people. Its name arose from the prominent, darkly coloured patches of decaying lymph glands found in the dying. The disease is bubonic plague, caused by a bacillus *Pasteurella pestis* and transmitted by the rat flea.

3 Pink disease This illness, known as acrodynia, occurred in infants and young children. It was typified by red swollen hands and feet and an aversion to light. It could last several months before recovery and was due to ingestion or contact with mercury.

4 Yellow fever This tropical disease is caused by a virus and is transmitted by mosquitoes. World travellers are familiar with the international precautions preventing its spread. The virus attacks the liver causing serious damage. Jaundice follows, tinging the tissues yellow. The Yellow Jack was the flag flown by vessels with yellow fever on board.

5 Black draught This old-fashioned purgative is primed for action. Its explosive mixture contains infusion of senna, Epsom salts, extract of liquorice and spirit of ammonia. These atomic ingredients look unpleasant and taste even worse. Dosage occurs at night – detonation follows in the morning.

6 Grey powder This uninspiring purge is seldom used today. It is composed of mercury and chalk; the chalk keeps the mercury in finely divided suspension. In this form, mercury dissolves slowly within the bowel and acts as an irritant on the muscular walls. Increased contractions follow with evacuation of the intestinal contents.

7 Blue blood Contrary to popular belief, the colour of one's blood is no indication of one's lineage nor exclusive ancestry. The idea arrived from Spain, where veins were more easily observed in the fair skins of the purely-bred than in those of Moorish descent. The blood's colour in duke or dustman reflects its degree of oxygenation.

8 Greenstick fracture A child's bones are immature and in breaking are likely to split rather than fracture cleanly. Often the break runs partly across the bone and then continues lengthwise. This process is reminiscent of a sapling broken in spring. For this reason it is termed a greenstick fracture.

9 White leg A mother recently delivered of her child may occasionally experience this unpleasant complication of obstetrics. It is characterized by a painful, swollen, white leg and indicates thrombosis in a deep leg vein. This condition requires immediate skilled treatment. Anticoagulant therapy is begun and may be combined with spinal injections.

10 Visual purple This substance is derived from vitamin A and is found in the retina – the photosensitive layer of the eye. When light rays strike the retina, visual purple is bleached. This reaction sets off nerve impulses which stream to the brain. Here they are coordinated and produce the remarkable phenomenon of vision.

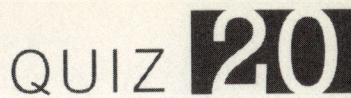

Which does what?

Good health is our greatest good fortune – yet what complexity of function this implies! Within our bodies so much goes on in so many places at the same time. Health is the integrated whole and herein lies the miracle of physiology.

Tissues, organs and secretions play highly specialized parts. But which does what? Can you name the chief function of these listed here?

1 White blood cell

2 Sweat

3 Lens of the eye

4 Bile

5 Red blood cell

6 Saliva

7 Wax of the ear

8 Spleen

9 Diaphragm

10 Fat

answers overleaf

1 Anti-invasion agents The white blood corpuscles provide an urgent and mobile defence for the body. Harmful invading organisms are seized and ingested by these haematological watchdogs – a process termed 'phagocytosis'. White cells congregate in enormous numbers in inflamed tissues. They form the chief component of pus.

2 Temperature regulation Sweat is principally a cooling device. Its evaporation from the body's surface removes heat from the skin and tends to lower the body's temperature. This process is continuous but normally passes unnoticed – so-called 'insensible perspiration'. In a minor capacity, sweating assists excretion by the body.

3 Fine focal adjustment The lens is the fine focal adjustment in the optical system of the eye. Most refraction of light takes place where the air is in contact with the front of the eye. By alteration of its shape, the elastic lens adjusts this refraction and by this means focusses the visual image sharply upon the retina.

4 Fat digestion Bile is secreted by the liver and is temporarily stored in the gall bladder. The bile salts emulsify fat. By lowering the surface tension, they prepare the fatty droplets for the action of digestive enzymes. Bile pigments are derived from broken down red blood cells. These pigments give bile its characteristic golden colour.

5 Oxygen transport Red blood cells carry oxygen from the lungs to the tissues of the body. Each is a tiny, flexible biconcave disc and is coloured by the pigment haemoglobin. Oxygen has a special affinity for this pigment. As the red cells recirculate back to the lungs, they assist in removing carbon dioxide from the tissues.

6 Lubricant of the mouth Saliva is the general lubricant of the mouth. Without it mastication would be difficult and speech would soon become impossible. The psychological aspects of its secretion are very apparent when contemplating a slice of lemon! Saliva contains the digestive enzyme ptyalin. This commences the breakdown of starch to sugar.

7 Protection The wax of the ear has a protective function. It is the hardened secretion of ceruminous glands which line the passageway down to the eardrum. Their sticky secretion traps particles of dust and discourages the entry of hopeful itinerant insects who chance to wander along.

8 Blood reservoir The spleen is found in the upper part of the abdomen on the left side. In times of need, its blood content may be added to the general circulation. Red blood cells, too old for further use, are broken down within its tissues. The spleen is not an essential organ and can be removed by surgical operation without ill-effect.

9 Respiration The diaphragm or midriff is a muscular dome, separating the thorax from the abdomen. On contraction and relaxation, its movements alternately inflate and deflate the lungs in the process of respiration. Breathing is supplemented by the muscles of the ribs. Variations of the diaphragm's normal contractions make laughing, sneezing and coughing possible.

10 Food storage Our fat is an enormous store of reserve food which we carry with us. Fat depots are located at strategic points throughout the tissues. The one situated just beneath the skin helps insulate the body and keep it warm. When times are hard, we live on our fat reserves and grow thin in the process.

QUIZ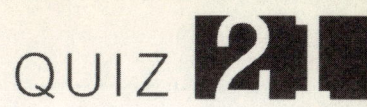

Spot the scope

Modern medical instruments are the greatest aid
to clinical investigations and accurage diagnosis.
Their evolution from early models to their gleaming,
present-day counterparts provides features of great
historical interest.

Ten 'tools for the job' form the answers to this
quiz. Each ends in 'scope'. Which 'scope' would be
used in examining the following?

1 The chest

2 The eye

3 The stomach

4 Bacteria

5 The bladder

6 The ear

7 The vocal cords

8 The bronchi of the lung

9 The nose

10 The lower bowel

answers overleaf

1 Stethoscope Familiar to everyone, this instrument has become the outward and visible sign of the medical man. It enables one to 'listen-in' to the body – a procedure technically known as 'auscultation'. Although the stethoscope finds its greatest use in examinations of the chest, it can be used with good effect on other parts of the body.

2 Ophthalmoscope The ophthalmoscope illuminates the inside of the eye and enables an examination of the retina to be made. This appears as a bright red background against which are seen the arteries, veins and optic disc. Retinal changes are liable to occur in many diseases and can be of great importance in diagnosis.

3 Gastroscope Gastroscopy is not a routine investigation but when employed can yield extremely valuable information in disease of the stomach. In the hands of an expert, the gastroscope is passed down the oesophagus and into the stomach, permitting a detailed inspection of the illuminated gastric interior.

4 Microscope The arrival of the microscope revolutionized medical thought. For the first time, it was possible to observe minute, living organisms, many of which were the agents of disease. Modern microscopy has become a highly complex science. The electron microscope has added its own quota of radical discoveries.

5 Cystoscope This ingenious surgical instrument has built-in lighting and telescopic systems. When passed into the bladder, a careful survey of the interior of this organ can be made. The openings of the ureters from right and left kidneys are seen and examined. Stones in the bladder will sometimes be viewed.

6 Auriscope The auriscope gives an excellent view of the eardrum, deep within the ear, which in health appears as a glistening pearl-grey membrane. It is invaluable in removing troublesome wax from the ear and in locating foreign bodies. These so readily find their way in, yet removal is quite a different story.

7 Laryngoscope The laryngoscope permits a rapid inspection of the larynx to be made. It has become an essential for the anaesthetist, whose constant duty is to maintain a clear airway from the lungs to the exterior of his unconscious patient. Respiratory obstruction can be rapidly located with this instrument and dealt with accordingly.

8 Bronchoscope This, like the gastroscope, is an instrument for the expert. It is passed through the larynx down into the trachea and enables an examination of the bronchi to be made. The procedure can supply conclusive evidence where diagnosis has been in doubt. Therapeutically, the bronchoscope plays a major part in the removal of inhaled foreign bodies.

9 Rhinoscope This instrument is first cousin to the auriscope and is used to illuminate and examine the interior of the nose. A common error is to imagine the nasal passages run upwards in the nose. In fact they do not but pass horizontally backwards to join the upper part of the throat.

10 Sigmoidoscope The sigmoidoscope enables a close scrutiny of the lower bowel lining to be made. It is inserted via the rectum and enters the sigmoid loop of the colon, which lies just above. The sigmoidoscope incorporates a lighting system and a small airpump. This latter inflates the lower bowel during passage of the instrument.

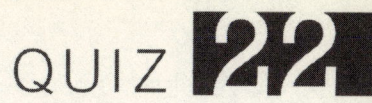

Artful adverts

To some people, life is an endless quest for that magical something which increases vigour, restores youth, guarantees health or enhances beauty. Obliging advertisers furnish suitable claims and, with a little applied psychology, everyone is happy.

How sound is your judgement in assessing these claims? Classify the examples given here as either fact or fantasy.

1 Common baldness can be cured.

2 Healthy bowels must be open once a day.

3 Adults can grow inches taller.

4 Glucose restores lost energy.

5 A truss will cure a rupture.

6 'Antiseptic' soaps kill the germs on our skins.

7 Everyone needs extra vitamins.

8 Cures can be bought for the common cold.

9 Stomach tablets are good for indigestion.

10 Tired? Listless? Jaded? What you need is a pep pill!

answers overleaf

1 No Medicine is still baffled by the problem of natural baldness. Hair creams and restorers have little effect. The condition commonly runs in families, affecting the male members. The different tendencies between men and women towards baldness are interesting and strongly suggest an underlying endocrinological cause.

2 No Bowel rhythms vary widely. Some function daily, others may open once a week. Each in its way can be normal and healthy. Preoccupation with one's bowels breeds much ill-health. If irregularities occur, most can be solved by exercise, regular habits and plenty of fruit and vegetables.

3 No Our height is determined by the length of our bones. During adolescence a period of active and rapid bone growth occurs with a corresponding increase in stature. This growing process burns itself out completely by the early twenties. It cannot be restarted and further growth in height as an adult is not possible.

4 Yes Glucose is rapidly assimilated by the body and provides an immediate source of energy. This sugar circulates freely in the blood and is readily available to the tissues. Excess can be stored by the liver for future needs. Glucose provides the food of the brain and is the fuel of muscular activity.

5 No Claims to cure rupture by wearing a truss are prominently displayed in magazines. Such appliances cannot cure and are merely palliative. With further time, the rupture worsens and the question of strangulation can arise. Ruptures are cured by a simple surgical operation. This should be considered at the earliest opportunity.

6 No Unattractively smelling soaps purporting to be used by doctors in their surgeries and surgeons in hospital are blessed with no special medicinal virtues. To obtain 'germ-free' hands, doctors scrub with a nailbrush for five minutes under running water. Any good quality soap is effective for this purpose.

7 No The indiscriminate swallowing of vitamins has become a pernicious fad. Enormous quantities of these synthetic products now disappear down British throats each year. A well-selected family diet will contain an adequate supply of natural vitamins for most needs. Extra should be taken on medical recommendation and not by random self-dosage.

8 No Although anticongestants may improve a blocked nose, the cold is a viral disease and in spite of intensive research no cure is yet forthcoming. Recovery depends on the natural resources of the body slowly overcoming the infection. This is best aided by keeping warm – if possible in bed. Most people have their favourite rituals when they feel a cold coming, but faith is here the greatest factor operating.

9 Yes Most indigestion tablets are extremely effective. There is nothing particularly complex in this. Digestive upsets so frequently result from an excess of the stomach's normal and natural acid secretion. The tablets are alkaline and neutralize the acidity. Pain disappears and the familiar sense of well-being returns once again.

10 No 'Pep pills' impart a temporary feeling of well-being – technically known as 'euphoria'. The effect is transient and is frequently followed by a corresponding phase of 'let down'. This in turn leads to taking more pills and the very real danger of habit formation. Medication of this kind requires the close supervision of a doctor.

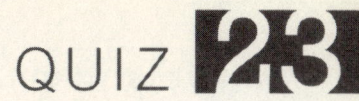

Something psychological

Psychology has long been a controversial subject. To some it appears as life's sweet secret of success, others decry it as the opium of the hopeless. In the hands of the hidden persuaders or motivational analysts, its power may be frightening particularly in an age when thinking for oneself, if not already vestigial, seems rapidly to be becoming inexcusable.

Few people today can afford to be ignorant of the basic principles of this powerful science. How much psychology do you know?

1 What do the letters IQ stand for?

2 Does sleep aid memory?

3 What is claustrophobia?

4 Can attention be divided?

5 What is the 'Rorschach test'?

6 Who introduced 'individual' psychology?

7 Which condition is characterized by compulsions to steal?

8 What is 'Aristotle's illusion'?

9 What was the mediaeval 'dancing madness'?

10 Can feelings be influenced by colour?

answers overleaf

1 Intelligence quotient This quotient is frequently used in psychology. By undergoing a series of tests, a person's 'mental age' can be assessed by comparing their score with standardized results. This 'mental age' is then divided by the person's real or 'chronological age' and the fraction is multiplied by 100 to give a percentage. An average IQ yields a percentage of approximately 100.

2 Yes A period of intensive study is best committed to memory if followed by a spell of mental inactivity — best of all by a period of sleep. Students should note that relaxation over coffee after a high-powered lecture may be done with the easiest of consciences and with full scientific approval.

3 Dread of enclosed spaces Claustrophobia is a morbid fear of enclosed spaces. This fear is generally experienced along with other symptoms of psychological illness. It should not be confused with feelings of uneasiness which many people have in underground trains or lifts. These feelings, though unpleasant, fall well within the limits of normality.

4 No Attention, surprisingly enough, cannot be divided. We attend to one thing at a time, although this — like a basket of fruit — may consist of several components. If we listen to a radio announcer and hold a conversation at the same time, our attention is alternating rapidly between the two. If we eat whilst watching television, we can do so because eating has become automatic and does not demand attention.

5 Ink-blot test This test is an aid to the assessment of personality. It consists of ten cards bearing ink-blot shapes, some of which are coloured. The subject undergoing testing views each card in turn and describes what the fantastic shapes suggest to him. His responses are noted and at a later stage are carefully analyzed.

6 Alfred Adler (1870–1937) This Austrian psychologist renounced the principles of psychoanalysis in 1911 and founded the School of Individual Psychology. He stressed the will to power was the dominant force in human life and that feelings of inferiority underlay the symptoms of neurosis.

7 Kleptomania Articles stolen by kleptomaniacs are quite often trivial and unimportant. The theft is commonly preceded by a great deal of pleasurable excitment, and afterwards remorse may be mixed with a sense of gratification. On being caught, petty thieves and shoplifters often put forward unwarranted pleas of kleptomania.

8 Illusion of doubling To demonstrate Aristotle's illusion, cross the index and middle fingers and place the tip of the nose between them. Rub the fingers gently up and down the nose, and 'two noses' will be clearly felt. This trick cheats our sense of perception. The brain interprets the stimuli as if the fingers were occupying their natural position.

9 Mass hysteria Historical outbreaks of dancing mania occurred in Europe during the troubled and turbulent Middle Ages. Begun by a few, the crazy antics of this fantastic dancing would spread like wildfire through the onlookers until hundreds could be involved. Individuals found themselves powerless to stop and eventually dropped to the ground in utter exhaustion, frequently foaming at the mouth.

10 Yes This phenomenon is technically known as 'chromaesthesia'. It can be observed in the colours we choose for our dress, home decoration and even motor car. It produces such expressions as 'cheerful reds', 'cool blues' and 'sombre greys'. Certain musicians perform at their best when bathed in light of their own personal colour.

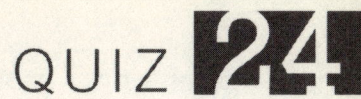

Skeleton in your cupboard

A skeleton could be viewed as the shape of things to come! 'What I am now, so you shall be!' Brrr — it doesn't bear thinking about too long; however, the grisliest skeletons often wear the widest grins and perhaps somewhere in this lies a moral for us all.

The best families keep skeletons in their cupboards. It is more than likely that you do too. You may be well familiar with it, but can you supply the information required here?

1 How many bones make up the skeleton?

2 Can the sex of a skeleton be determined?

3 Can a bone be tied in a knot?

4 What is bone marrow?

5 Do we possess tail bones?

6 Is there a bone in the throat?

7 Are wrist bones found in a newborn child?

8 Which bone looks like a bat in flight?

9 Can horsemen develop a special bone of their own?

10 What are the bones of the ear?

answers overleaf

1 206 This is the figure usually quoted but it can easily vary. Sometimes two bones may fuse in the skeleton or one bone can exist in two or more parts. These variations are not necessarily pathological. X-ray photography has shown quite wide variations to exist in normal, healthy people.

2 Yes This is most easily seen by the pelvis. A woman's pelvis is adapted for childbearing and shows well-marked characteristics. Most easily identified is the angle between the pubic bones at the front. In the female this angle is wide and approximately 90 degrees. In the male the sub-pubic angle is narrow and not more than 70 degrees.

3 Yes A bone treated with acid will lose its inorganic salts but still retain its general shape. These salts confer the bone's rigidity. The organic tissues remain and are elastic, enabling a suitable long bone to be bent into a circle or even tied in a knot.

4 Blood-forming tissue Bone marrow is the organ which manufactures blood. Both red and white corpuscles are made here. All the bones of a young child are filled with active blood-producing marrow. In the adult, however, fat replaces the marrow of the limb bones and active marrow persists only in such bones as the sternum, vertebrae and hip.

5 Yes Four small bones are fused at the base of the spine to form the coccyx. This is the remnant of man's tail. At an early embryological stage, a human tail is very evident but disappears with further development. The coccyx remains – and reminds some of us of our ancestry.

6 Yes This is the 'U-shaped' hyoid bone, found just above the larynx in the neck. The Greek orator Demosthenes once successfully evaded a public speech by pleading he 'had a bone in his throat'! The hyoid bone is freely movable and is retained in position by its muscular attachments.

7 No The wrists of a newborn child are purely cartilaginous. No bone has yet formed and on X-ray the wrists show as two curious gaps. The bones are still in no hurry to appear during childhood. Ossification proceeds very gradually and the last bone does not form until the child is approximately 13 years old.

8 Sphenoid bone This bone is found behind the eyes at the base of the brain. When isolated, its bat-like appearance is quite uncanny. The outspread wings support lobes of the brain; its body contains the 'turkish saddle' which houses the all-important pituitary gland.

9 Yes Equestrians of long-standing – old cavalrymen, postillions, cowboys – may develop a small extra bone of their own. This is the 'rider's bone' – a centre of ossification which appears among the muscles at the inner side of the thigh. These muscular tissues are damaged by prolonged rough treatment in the saddle and react to the situation by forming bone.

10 Hammer, anvil and stirrup These are the three tiny bones of the ear. Each is named from its extraordinary appearance. These ossicles span the middle compartment of the ear and transmit vibrations from the eardrum. They function as a miniature lever which concentrates and greatly increases the force of the sound waves.

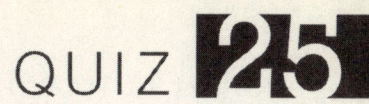
Magic and mysticism

Medicine, like time, continually progresses. Earlier procedures, performed in the name of healing, may horrify us now and make our blood run cold. Former beliefs may now make us smile, yet in their time were sincerely held with a view to relieving suffering. The blessings of the twentieth century are sometimes doubted – but in the clinical field are indisputable.

These older ideas form an odd collection. How much of this quiz can you answer?

1 Which operation was performed to release demons from the head?

2 Who cured by 'animal magnetism'?

3 What does the symbol ℞ stand for?

4 Which disease was called the 'king's evil'?

5 Did the Greeks use snakes medicinally?

6 Which medicinal plant 'shrieked on being uprooted'?

7 What was the 'sacred disease'?

8 Who introduced phrenology?

9 Which jewel was thought to prevent drunkeness?

10 Are love philtres effective?

answers overleaf

1 Trephining This operation consists of making a hole in the vault of the skull. Strangely enough, it has been carried out among primitive peoples since prehistoric times. Their concept of so many diseases, from headaches to insanity, was the notion of 'demons in the head'. The hole was made to let the demons escape!

2 Franz Mesmer Mesmer established his sensational practice in Paris in 1778. He claimed to cure by his own special powers of 'animal magnetism'. Inundated with patients, he extended his treatment en masse by using 'magnetized water'. Mesmer's methods were the forerunner of hypnotism. His name is immortalized in our expression to 'mesmerize'.

3 Recipe This is latin for 'take' and its abbreviation is found at the head of every prescription. The tail of the Rwill be seen to have a stroke through it. It is said that this symbol really represents the sign of Jupiter (♃). At one time, this deity was invoked to bless all prescriptions. On occasion, his intervention appears to have been a dire necessity!

4 Scrofula This is a tuberculous condition of the neck in which the glands are badly affected. For centuries it was believed to be curable by the touch of the monarch and was consequently known as 'king's evil'. A hard-working monarch would touch thousands in a year. In England, the practice ceased after the death of Queen Anne.

5 Yes In the Temples of Healing of Ancient Greece, harmless snakes were employed to lick the eyes and sores of the afflicted who came for treatment. These temples were sacred to Aesculapius, the God of Medicine. Miraculous cures followed visitations from this god whilst the patient slept.

6 Mandrake Accounts of mandrake are found in ancient herbals. Its roots were visualized as human figures. The plant was believed to scream on being uprooted, turning insane anyone within earshot. A recommended method of collection was to tie the plant to a dog. Mandrake itself was used as a sedative.

7 Epilepsy Ancient ignorance attributed epilepsy to the displeasure of the Gods. It was accordingly known as the 'sacred disease'. Hippocrates, the outstanding Greek physician to whom so much is owed, rigorously opposed this idea. He taught that epilepsy had a natural cause and should in no way be thought a divine affliction.

8 Franz Gall Phrenology claimed that the shape of the skull determined mental characteristics. It was introduced by Gall at the end of the eighteenth century. 'Bump reading' soon leapt into fashion. Its wonderful charts of the head are still to be found at fairgrounds and with fortune-tellers.

9 Amethyst This attractive purple stone is a variety of quartz. It was held in high esteem by the ancients who believed it to be a charm against intoxication. If worn or dropped into the wine, its protection was secured. For knock-out concoctions, the drinking vessel itself was sometimes made of amethyst.

10 No Love philtres, like faint hearts, never won fair lady, yet their sale has been popular down through the ages in all parts of the world. Even today odd cases still arise. Wooing by alchemy is doomed to failure. Sad though it may be, the love philtre is wishful thinking and has no realistic basis.

Medical Knowledge for Fun

What the doctor ordered

Patients so often feel they know exactly what is needed. 'Just give me a drop of the stuff you take yourself, Doctor!' Prescribing is by means so simple, and one man's physic may well prove another man's flatulence.

A doctor might order anything in the list given here in the interests of his patients' health. What are the items? What is he really after?

1 Barium meal

2 Haemoglobin estimation

3 Lumbar puncture

4 Spiritus vini galli

5 White blood count

6 Intravenous pyelogram

7 ESR

8 Hirudo medicinalis

9 Mantoux test

10 Sternal puncture

answers overleaf

1 Stomach X-ray The stomach, like other muscular tissues, does not show well on a straightforward X-ray. The difficulty is solved by the patient drinking some 'barium cream'. This viscid paste is opaque to X-rays and by filling the stomach allows the shape and movements of this organ to be clearly seen.

2 Routine anaemia test Haemoglobin is the pigment of the red blood cells and confers on blood its characteristic colour. By using a refined technique, a haemoglobin estimation really compares the 'redness' of a patient's blood with an accepted standard for normal. Normality is taken as 100%. Values considerably short of this indicate anaemia.

3 Specimen of cerebrospinal fluid A specimen of this fluid which bathes the brain and spinal cord can be obtained by passing a suitable needle between the lower lumbar vertebrae. Analysis of it yields valuable information on the state of the central nervous system, and plays a vital part in the correct diagnosis of neurological illness.

4 Brandy This spirit is prepared by distilling wine and contains approximately 40% alcohol. Its carminative action upon the stomach reduces flatulence and finds a great demand at multi-course dinners. Brandy imparts a feeling of warmth to the body by dilating the blood vessels of the skin. Taken last thing at night, it induces sleep.

5 White corpuscle count Much can be told of a patient's condition by counting and examining the white corpuscles of the blood. Normally, 5000 to 10 000 of these are found in each cubic millimetre of blood. Their total number and their type vary considerably with disease. Increases occur with infections and some blood disorders. Decreases are found in starvation and after the administration of certain drugs.

6 Kidney X-ray For normal X-ray purposes, the kidney can be outlined by a simple injection of radio-opaque dye given into a vein of the arm. The kidney removes this dye from the blood, concentrates it and passes it into the upper end of the ureter.

An X-ray film taken at this point will allow both kidney and ureter to be clearly visualized.

7 Erythrocyte sedimentation rate In some of the chronic diseases, progress can best be followed by observing the rate at which red blood cells (erythrocytes) settle out from their plasma. Prepared specimens of blood are set vertically in narrow glass tubes and the distance the cells have settled in one hour is measured in millimetres. Increased rates of sedimentation accompany the active stages of tuberculosis, rheumatoid arthritis and cancer.

8 The medicinal leech Only the strongest-minded physicians prescribe – and get – leeches today. In earlier times, the use of these revolting little creatures was all too frequent. This was the era of 'bleeding' and a blood loss of approximately half an ounce per leech could be reckoned. Leeches secrete a special anticoagulant which prevents the blood from clotting as they drink.

9 Tuberculosis sensitivity test For the Mantoux test, a purified extract of tubercle bacilli is injected into the skin. Most healthy adults carry within them an old inactive tuberculous focus and accordingly react positively, with a localized area of inflammation at the site of the injection. Healthy infants should be insensitive to this test and react negatively. A positive result in an infant is suggestive of active tuberculosis.

10 Bone marrow examination An examination of bone marrow can yield vital information in certain anaemias and other disorders of the blood. The specimen is conveniently obtained from the sternum or breast bone, using a syringe and wide-bore needle. The marrow is spread as a thin film on a glass slide and, after staining, is examined microscopically.

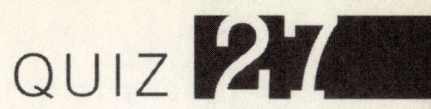
Art and affliction

It is uncanny how illness and suffering have dogged so many of the world's finest creative artists. Is this coincidental – or can some deeper link be found? Is the artist any less fitted for the physical rigours of this life, or is, in fact, his inspiration drawn from the experience of his own suffering? Artists differ, and no generalization can be made.

The following persons are renowned in the arts. Each was afflicted – you are asked to say how.

1 John Keats

2 Vincent Van Gogh

3 Homer

4 Henri Toulouse-Lautrec

5 Ludwig van Beethoven

6 Sergei Rachmaninov

7 Demosthenes

8 Sir Arthur Sullivan

9 Maurice Utrillo

10 Frédéric Chopin

answers overleaf

1 Tuberculosis Keats, oddly enough, embarked on a medical career. He served his apprenticeship with a surgeon and later became a dresser at Guy's Hospital. He then gave up surgery, devoting himself to his poetry. Advanced tuberculosis destroyed his health and he died, shortly after his arrival in Italy, a young man of twenty-five years.

2 Insanity Among Van Gogh's greatest paintings were those made during his tempestuous years in the asylum of Saint-Rémy. These epitomize the tormented passions and emotional chaos he was experiencing at this time. In one outburst, he cut off his own ear. Later, he ended his life by shooting himself.

3 Blindness The facts of Homer's life history have been lost in antiquity. Critics have argued his very existence. Legend affirms that Homer was blind. Blindness can inspire outstanding creative ability. Compensation by the remaining senses appears to promote a heightened sense of beauty and to increase the depth of understanding.

4 Deformed legs As a boy, Toulouse-Lautrec's growth was stunted by fractures of both legs. He grew up a grotesque, dwarf-like cripple. The bitter frustration of his physical deformities sought outlet in his paintings. Horses at full gallop and dancers with powerful well-proportioned legs personified the movement and action which fate had denied to the artist himself.

5 Deafness Beethoven's tragic deafness had become obvious by the age of thirty. It followed an infection in his earlier years. In the face of this terrible handicap, his spirit remained indomitable. His musical genius drew inspiration from his affliction and produced those masterpieces which others – but not himself – would hear.

6 Melancholia Rachmaninov's recurrent attacks of sustained and morbid gloom inspired his finest compositions. The intensity of these moods can be appreciated on listening to his music. In one prolonged depressive illness he became convinced he would never write again. On recovery, he composed the magnificent Second Piano Concerto and dedicated it to his physician.

7 Stammer The brilliant Greek orator Demosthenes is said to have overcome his stammer by practising with pebbles in his mouth. He often rehearsed his speeches on the seashore, making his voice resound over and above the noise of the waves. Stammering has many causes. Treatment should be started as early as possible.

8 Renal calculus Sullivan suffered greatly from a stone in his kidney. Among his finest and most touching melodies, were those composed between bouts of renal colic. The intensity of these attacks can be extreme. The emotional relief on remission of the pain would lend itself well to expression by music.

9 Alcoholism The French artist Utrillo was an alcoholic. As a child he was given wine and water to keep him quiet. By boyhood his craving for drink was well-established. His life of painting was punctuated by his drinking bouts and hospital admissions. He showed little response to any treatment and his alcoholic cravings persisted to the end.

10 Tuberculosis Chopin was consumptive. His health and life were destroyed by tuberculosis of the lung. From this bleak background emerged music of exquisite beauty. His sufferings were greatly mitigated by the care of George Sand, who did much to prolong the composer's life. A quarrel separated them and two years later Chopin died in Paris.

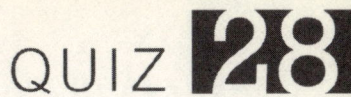
Cope with the crisis

Accidents happen and emergencies arise – usually at the most inconvenient moments. On these occasions, a little knowledge of the right kind can save time, trouble and sometimes even life.

Ten 'crises' are set out on the left below. Their solutions are mixed in the right-hand column. Can you cope with each crisis, selecting the appropriate answer from the right for each of these emergencies?

1 A troublesome flea		A wisp of cotton wool
2 A tight ring stuck on the finger		Warm olive oil
3 A bee sting		A cold compress
4 Obstinate bleeding from a minor cut		Mustard and water
5 An insect in the ear		Head between the knees
6 A fish-hook in the flesh		A piece of string
7 A child believed to have eaten poisonous berries		Gargle with vinegar
8 A 'black eye'		Some sodium bicarbonate
9 A threatened faint		A white blanket
10 A fish bone in the throat		A pair of pliers

answers overleaf

1 A white blanket To catch the flea, spread the blanket on the floor. Stand in the middle and carefully undress. When uncovered, the flea will jump and land trapped among the white wool fibres, showing up clearly. Easy disposal can now be effected by pressing a damp tablet of soap firmly on the flea.

2 A piece of string Wind the string tightly round and round the finger from its tip down as far as the ring. Now slip the string through the ring and pull gently back towards the finger-tip. The string unwinds and gradually removes the ring from the finger.

3 Some sodium bicarbonate Bee stings are acidic and may be neutralized with some sodium bicarbonate or ammonia. First remove the sting which the bee leaves behind. Wasp venom is alkaline and can be treated with vinegar or lemon juice. Wasps do not leave their stings behind. If available, antihistamine cream is excellent for both types of sting.

4 A wisp of cotton wool Obstinate bleeding from a minor cut can frequently be arrested by placing a wisp of cotton wool over the wound. To avoid infection, this cotton wool must be surgically clean. The enormous number of fibres greatly increases the area of clotting activity and the bleeding area is soon effectively sealed off.

5 Warm olive oil The removal of an insect from the ear is quite simple if properly done. The patient should lie on their side with the affected ear uppermost. By running warm olive oil gently into the ear until full, the insect will float to the top and can be easily captured.

6 A pair of pliers On account of its barb, a fish-hook in the flesh cannot be withdrawn along its route of entry. It must be gradually worked onwards until both barb and point have re-emerged through the skin. If these are now snipped off, the blunt shaft of the hook can be easily removed.

7 Mustard and water The essential thing here is to make the child sick. Mustard and water is an effective emetic, using one tablespoon of mustard to a tumblerful of water. If any berries can be preserved for identification, so much the better. Medical aid must be sought immediately.

8 A cold compress A 'black eye' should be treated with a cold compress for the first twenty-four hours. This is soothing and minimizes the resultant degree of bruising. On removing the compress, treatment is continued by bathing the bruised area with warm water. The old-fashioned beefsteak can claim no advantage over treatment by the cold compress.

9 Head between the knees A faint threatens when too little blood is circulating to the brain. Getting the head between the knees will ,in most cases, solve the problem. If consciousness is lost, the patient should be laid flat on their back with the legs slightly raised. Loosen clothing around the neck. Consciousness should return within a few minutes.

10 Gargle with vinegar A fine fish bone stuck in the throat may resist all attempts to shift it, and for a time can be extremely distressing. On these occasions, it is worth gargling with some vinegar. Vinegar, as a weak acid, helps dissolve the bone. This combined with the gargling may be just enough to effect dislodgement.

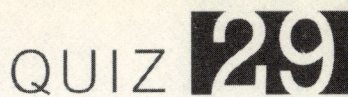

Clinical judgement

Cases arise in forensic medicine against which the best of detective fiction may appear surprisingly tame. While doctors argue and solicitors pontificate, the learned professions of law and medicine combine their talents in the field of jurisprudence.

This quiz devotes itself to medico-legal problems. Answers, please, to the cross-examination.

1 Can an insane person make a valid will?

2 What is dactylography?

3 Must a special death certificate be obtained for cremation?

4 What is 'policeman's disease'?

5 Can paternity be proven by laboratory examination?

6 Which officer of the Crown must investigate unexplained death?

7 What standard of eyesight is required for a driving licence?

8 Is a poison defined by law?

9 What is 'rigor mortis'?

10 Can drunkenness be accurately assessed by blood tests?

answers overleaf

1 Yes To make a valid will, the law merely requires a person to be of 'sound disposing mind'. This, in effect, means that the testator shall know what he possesses, to whom he can reasonably bequeath it, and shall have a good reason for disposing of his property in this way. It is quite possible for a sound will to be made by an insane person.

2 Study of fingerprints Our fingerprints are personal and exclusive. No two persons in the world can have the same. Their pattern throughout our lives remains unchanged and attempts to destroy them by damaging the skin are quite unsuccessful. The skin regrows and the fingerprints again emerge with the full detail of their original pattern.

3 Yes For the purpose of cremation, two doctors are required to examine the body and issue a second, more detailed death certificate. The doctors may not be partners or related to each other. The first will have been in attendance during the final illness, and the second must have qualified in medicine not less than five years previously.

4 Metatarsalgia Pain from the metatarsal bones of the feet may develop in heavy persons subjected to long periods of standing. Ligaments between the bones become stretched and excessive pressure falls on the underlying nerves. With metatarsalgia, the policeman's lot is anything but a happy one.

5 Yes In earlier times, blood-grouping could only determine who the father wasn't. Today, with DNA examination from white blood cells, spermatozoa or buccal scrapings, paternity can be identified accurately.

6 The coroner English law requires the coroner to inquire into any violent, suspicious or unexplained death. Deaths occurring in prisons or asylums must also be brought to the coroner's notice. Coroners' inquiries are made in matters relating to the removal of dead bodies from England and perhaps most picturesquely of all, in matters covering treasure trove.

7 Ability to read a number plate at 25 yards Before issue of a driving licence, applicants are required to prove that they can read, with glasses if necessary, a vehicle numberplate at a distance of 25 yards. The test should be carried out in good daylight and the number plate must contain six letters and figures.

8 No The control of poisons is governed by many Acts, Rules, Schedules and Regulations. It may seem remarkable that with this vast amount of legislation, the law does not in fact define a poison. In practice, it is accepted that any substance causing harm to the body when taken internally or applied externally, falls into this category.

9 Cadaveric rigidity The stiffening which occurs in a body fairly soon after death is due to coagulation of the muscle proteins by lactic acid. It normally lasts for some twelve to eighteen hours before disappearing once again. Rigor mortis can sometimes have a medico-legal value when an assessment is being made of the time at which death occurred.

10 No Individuals vary quite widely in response to standard concentrations of alcohol in the blood. Extreme values are compatible with sobriety or drunkenness – but this fact would be obvious anyway. The effects of more intermediate values cannot be predicted with accuracy for any one person, and a knowledge of such values by themselves could not establish a state of drunkenness. However, the legal limits for alcohol if driving are 80 milligrams per 100 millilitres of blood or 35 micrograms per 100 millilitres of breath. If driving, it is far better to abstain completely from drinking.

Vital statistics

The current widespread interest in human figures can scarcely be confused with a universal yearning for arithmetic. Answers to problems of reduction and proportion are regularly sought in doctors' consulting rooms. For all that, the statistics of our bodies make compulsive reading.

Can you say...

1 How many Calories are needed each day by the average working man?

2 How many hairs are on the head?

3 How many different tastes we can appreciate?

4 How much blood do we have?

5 What is the fastest rate at which nerve impulses travel?

6 How many bones make up the backbone?

7 What is the frequency range of the human ear?

8 How many arches are found in each foot?

9 How many milk teeth do we have?

10 How many times is blood thicker than water?

answers overleaf

1 3000 The Calorie is the physiological unit of energy. In twenty-four hours, the 'average working man' requires approximately 3000. These Calories are supplied each day in our food. Excessive intake, over and above requirement, leads to an increase in weight. Slimming has become the art of low-calorie diets.

2 100 000 The number of hairs on the head has been calculated to be in the region of 100 000. Human hair is classified into three types – exemplified by the Mongol, the European and the African. The differences are explained in terms of the shape of the hair in cross-section. The flatter the section, the more easily the hair curls.

3 Four Strange as it may seem, we are able to recognize only four different qualities in taste. These are bitter, sweet, salt and sour. Most of what we normally call taste is, in fact, smell. If this faculty is removed – as frequently happens with a bad head cold – we realize just how limited our true sense of taste really is.

4 11 pints Blood is a well-adapted, multipurpose fluid. It supplies food and oxygen to the body's tissues and at the same time removes their waste products. Its white cells and antibodies are constantly warding off infection. By clotting, blood seals off any leak in the circulation and provides the essential first stage in wound healing.

5 120 Metres per second Some nerve impulses travel with lightning-like rapidity within the body. Their speeds are related to the thickness of the nerve fibre along which they are travelling. Top speeds occur in the thickest fibres and can reach 120 metres per second.

6 33 Our backbone (vertebral column) consists of 33 individual bones. It its these that permit such extensive movements of the body. They include seven cervical (neck), 12 thoracic (back), five lumbar (loins), five fused sacral and five fused caudal vertebrae – fused to form the coccyx or man's rudimentary tail.

7 16 to 20 000 vibrations per second This range of frequency is usually quoted for the human ear. It is an approximate one and shows marked individual variation. The lowest frequencies are sometimes heard as the deepest notes from a large organ. The highest frequencies are found in the squeak of a bat. Some adolescents, but not adults, can appreciate the extreme upper range of the frequency scale.

8 Three The foot has three arches – two run lengthwise and one runs crosswise. The arches are held up by the bones, ligaments and muscles. These supports are susceptible to prolonged strain, particularly that which comes from excessive standing. If the arches weaken, a flat foot results.

9 20 A child's full 'milk set' contains 20 teeth – 12 less than the adult quota. In each jaw there are four incisors, two canines and four molars. These teeth are shed during childhood by a process of root absorption. No premolars are found among the milk teeth.

10 Five times At body temperature, human blood is approximately five times as thick as water. This increased viscosity is mostly due to the large numbers of red and white corpuscles suspended within the plasma. To a lesser extent, the blood platelets – concerned in clotting – and the proteins of the serum make their own contribution towards the greater viscosity of blood.

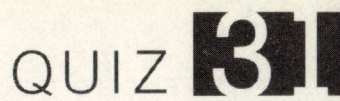

Medical Knowledge for Fun

Tinker, tailor...

When in doubt, blame the work! Yet this much maligned pastime is an essential for any healthy and satisfying life. Too frequently troubles start when the point of retirement is reached.

In this quiz, things are very much the wrong way around. In each case, the occupation has caused the illness. Can you say what is...?

1 Stoker's cramp

2 Chauffeur's fracture

3 Knifegrinder's rot

4 Painter's colic

5 Butcher's wart

6 Diver's cramp

7 Hatter's shakes

8 Housemaid's knee

9 Woolsorter's disease

10 Film star's eye

answers overleaf

1 Progressive salt loss Stoker's cramp is an example of a salt depletion. Sweat contains salt and excessive sweating can mean a heavy salt loss. Thirsty stokers who drink plain water are liable to develop muscular cramps. They are replacing fluid but not salt. Salt added to the drinking water cures the symptoms.

2 Backfire fracture Here the radius is broken, usually just above the wrist. It follows the unwary cranking of a motor car. A backfire from the engine can kick back the starting handle, fracturing the radius by a sudden hyperextension of the wrist. Caution is always necessary cranking a powerful car.

3 Siderosis This is a dust disease of the lungs caused by the inhalation of minute steel particles – traditionally in the practice of knife and scissor grinding. The steel dust is highly irritant and sets up inflammatory changes. Healthy lung tissue is relentlessly replaced by dense fibrous scars and becomes the breeding ground for major respiratory infection.

4 Lead poisoning Intense abdominal cramps are a feature of chronic lead poisoning. Anaemia also occurs and a blue line of lead sulphide can sometimes be found on the gums. Painters absorbed the lead from their paints and were subsequently seized with intestinal colic. The conditions of workers in contact with lead are now controlled by Act of Parliament.

5 Cutaneous tuberculosis Butchers were liable to find warty growths appearing on their fingers, hands or arms. These excrescences followed the direct implantation of tuberculosis bacteria. The bacteria came from infected meat and found a ready entrance in the cracked hands and fingers of the butcher.

6 Decompression sickness Muscular pains, known as 'the bends', develop in divers who surface too quickly after working at high underwater pressures. The sudden reduction of pressure releases nitrogen gas from the blood and the bubbles formed rapidly clog the tissues. This sets up acute muscular pain and in severe cases will cause paralysis.

7 Mercurial palsy Mercury is used in the felting of hats. Its prolonged and indiscriminate use is liable to affect the nervous system, causing the 'hatter's shakes'. This is mercurial palsy – a consequence of chronic mercury poisoning. It appears as a fine trembling of the muscles of the face, tongue and limbs. This was the basis of the 'Mad Hatter' in Lewis Carroll's *Alice in Wonderland*.

8 Prepatellar bursitis In housemaid's knee, a small sac (bursa) found just in front of the kneecap is inflamed and distended with fluid. The diagnosis is unmistakable and the cause usually lies in prolonged kneeling on hard surfaces. Clergyman's knee is also recognized; here an identical swelling occurs just below the knee.

9 Anthrax of the lung The highest incidence of this disease fell among those working in woolsorting and brushmaking. Imported wool, hair and hides were frequently infected and carried anthrax spores. These were inhaled by the workers and gave rise to a pneumonia which ran a rapidly fatal course. The importation of wool, hair and hides is nowadays rigorously controlled.

10 Ultraviolet conjunctivitis Injudicious film stars may find themselves with acutely inflamed and painful eyes. The cause lies with the ultraviolet light which emanates from the brilliant electric lamps on the set. Similiar trouble can be caused by bright sunlight reflected from snow. For this reason, the wearing of sunglasses whilst winter sporting is a wise precaution.

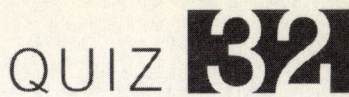

Hysteria most horrible

The history of witchcraft is the story of hysteria. This medical phenomenon can be found both on an individual or mass basis. Mass hysteria is liable to erupt when the stability of a country is in jeopardy. It has always had a very close linkage with witchcraft. Hysteria is one of the most baffling conditions of medicine. Individually, almost any symptom known to us can be simulated by a person suffering from hysteria.

How much of the following can you answer?

1 Which centuries saw the mass hysterical persecutions at their worst in England?

2 What was the water test for a witch?

3 What is 'globus hystericus'?

4 Which king wrote *Daemonologie*?

5 What are 'devil's seals'?

6 What were 'witches familiars'?

7 What was 'arcus eroticus'?

8 What are the 'stigmata'?

9 Who was the Witchfinder General?

10 What is hysterical aphonia?

answers overleaf

1 16th and 17th Centuries Despite an Act outlawing witchcraft having been passed in 1542, during the reign of Henry VIII, it was during the period of intense political and religious unrest in the reign of Elizabeth I that the persecution of witches reached the degree of mass hysteria. Hundreds of women were tortured and unjustly put to death on trumped-up accusations. This practice continued well into the 17th Century.

2 Swimming a witch With hands bound and tied to feet, a suspected witch was flung into deep water. If she floated this was taken as a positive sign of witchcraft since the water had rejected her. If she sank, the sign was negative, though in this case the poor woman was in imminent danger of death from drowning.

3 Lump in the throat Globus hystericus is a medical symptom whereby a sizeable lump is felt in the throat and is capable of moving up and down. No lump as such exists and physical examination reveals nothing. The sensation is due to an increased tension in the pharyngeal muscles.

4 James I (1566–1625) King James I of England and VI of Scotland published his work _Daemonologie_ in 1597. He advocated the 'swimming' of suspected witches and also believed they could be identified by significant external marks on the body. This led to the stripping and searching and most wrongful condemnation of innumerable innocent victims.

5 Patches of anaesthesia In hysterical patients, local patches of anaesthesia can be found where pain is absent and pins and needles can be pushed through the skin with impunity. These, in the searches for witches, were known as devil's seals and were enough to condemn a suspected witch. In some patients, whole areas of anaesthesia corresponding to a long glove or stocking can be found. These bear no correspondence to the distribution of cutaneous sensory nerves.

6 Imps These formed the various army of low-ranking demons in the shape of cats, rats, toads, weasles, mice and other creatures, which attended witches and advised them on their malicious activities. The witch was believed to suckle these imps and give of her blood to them.

7 Arched back This condition could be found typically in convents and abbeys where hysterical nuns in bed would believe themselves being raped by Satan. The back would contract separating from the bed and form an involuntary arc between the head and the pelvis.

8 Signs of Christ's wounds A further manifestation of hysteria can be found in the curious phenomenon of the appearance in hands, feet and side of red patches simulating the wounds of Christ. In earlier times, such individuals were scorned or discredited by the Church authorities.

9 Matthew Hopkins This loathsome individual plied his obscene trade in 1645. He was a failed lawyer of Ipswich who settled in Manningtree, Essex. East Anglia was an area where the hysteria of witchcraft was particularly prevalent. He went about denouncing and torturing hundreds of innocent women as witches and sent them to the gallows. He was well paid for each 'witch' that he arraigned and he engineered mass trials of these simple unfortunate women.

10 Loss of voice It is possible for a hysterical patient to be literally struck dumb. Again, no organic cause exists for this. Hysterics are notoriously suggestible and sometimes an authoritarian statement that speech will return at a specific time on a specific day will be totally effective in the return of the voice.

Roman posers

The well-timed Latin tag, adroitly culled like a conjurer's rabbit from the hat, has rescued many a medical man in moments of uncertainty. With minimum knowledge came maximum effect and where the patient recovered who could complain?

Now is your chance of a *quid pro quo*. Each term below has an interesting Latin origin – but what did each originally mean?

1 Muscle

2 Acetabulum

3 Pupil

4 Sartorius

5 Calculus

6 Shingles

7 Cancer

8 Insulin

9 Carbuncle

10 Fibula

answers overleaf

1 A little mouse Latin *musculus* is 'a little mouse'. Why was this term chosen for the body's contractile organs? It is difficult to be absolutely certain. Some have said that a muscle with its tendon suggests a mouse and its tail. Another theory maintains that rippling muscles beneath the skin suggest a small mouse running under a blanket!

2 A vinegar cup The acetabulum is the deep socket of the hip joint. In Latin, its name means 'a vinegar cup'. Articulation with the spherical head of the femur forms a joint of unrivalled stability. Occasionally, the acetabulum may fail to develop properly. This causes congenital dislocation of the hip.

3 A little doll Latin *pupilla* is 'a little doll'. Gaze closely into another's eye and you will see a living, miniature replica of yourself set against a black background. This is the tiny 'doll' whose name in medicine has come to denote the central black aperture of the eye itself.

4 A tailor Latin *sartorius* is 'the tailor' and is the name of the long, slender muscle which runs diagonally across the thigh downwards and inwards from the hip. This muscle ends just below the knee. On its contraction the leg is moved to the classical position of the cross-legged tailor.

5 A pebble Latin *calculus* is 'a pebble'. Ancient reckoning by pebbles gave us the English word 'calculate'. Calculi may form in many parts of the body. Most, but not all, show up on X-ray and if necessary can be removed surgically. The lithotomists of earlier centuries travelled the country 'cutting for the stone'.

6 A girdle Shingles is a corruption of the latin *cingulum* meaning 'a girdle'. It is the disease of the Herpes zoster virus. The girdle is formed by the rows of small blisters which creep slowly round the body wall. Chickenpox, strangely enough, is caused by the same virus.

7 A crab Latin *cancer* is 'a crab' – as followers of horoscopes will already know. Since the earliest times, this disease has plagued mankind and its final conquest is still eagerly awaited. The ancients noted the changes which can occur in the appearance of the veins and likened these to the limbs of a crab.

8 An island Latin *insula* is 'an island'. Set deep within the tissues of the pancreas gland are countless microscopic groups of special cells. These are the important islets of Langerhans, whose secretion has been named insulin. Insulin is a hormone, essential for normal sugar metabolism. Deficiency of insulin leads to diabetes.

9 A burning coal Latin *carbunculus* is 'a piece of burning coal' – a fact well appreciated by those with first-hand experience of this condition. The carbuncle occurs with a staphylococcal invasion of the subcutaneous tissues, and erupts like a cluster of closely-packed boils. The condition is extremely distressing and in certain sites is highly dangerous.

10 A brooch pin The fibula is the slender bone found on the outer side of the lower leg. It is subsidiary to the tibia or shinbone, which takes the full weight of the body. Latin *fibula* is 'a brooch pin'. This remarkable similarity is at once evident when the tibia and fibula are viewed together in their natural positions.

Greek teasers

Greek ingenuity for the appropriate word is as legendary as the exploits of Odysseus. Greek influence in medicine has provided a wealth of interesting terms, often with unexpected derivations.

The words here have interesting Greek origins. What does each word really mean?

1 Poliomyelitis

2 Clinic

3 Psychosomatic

4 Surgeon

5 Melancholia

6 Hypochondriac

7 Enzyme

8 Hermaphrodite

9 Migraine

10 Staphylococcus

answers overleaf

1 Inflammation of the grey marrow Several Greek words are involved here. *Polio* means 'grey', *myelos* 'marrow', and -*itis* denotes an 'inflammation'. Poliomyelitis is otherwise known as infantile paralysis. Nerve cells in the grey matter of the spinal cord are inflamed by attacking viruses. These cells control muscular movements and their damage precedes the tragic paralyses.

2 A bed Greek *kline* is 'a bed'. The advantages of bed need no elaboration; these are only too apparent when the alarm clock rings on a typical winter's morning. Centuries of illness have proved bed-rest to be of prime importance in healing disease and the bedside has become the recognized seat for medical practice.

3 Mind-body The Greek *psyche* implies 'the mind' and *soma* is 'the body'. Modern medicine recognizes that many physical ailments can be caused or aggravated by adverse mental factors. To this aspect of disease the term psychosomatic has been applied. There is of course no natural division between the mind and body and their harmonious interaction is essential to any good health.

4 A handworker The Greek *cheir* is 'the hand' and *ergon* is 'work', but the skill of the modern surgeon has evolved far beyond mere manual dexterity. Facilities are available to him from so many scientific fields. It is the surgeon's high standard of technical knowledge which enables him to place these at the disposal of his patients.

5 Black bile In Greek, *melas* means 'black' and *chole* is 'bile'. This extraordinary derivation is steeped in antiquity and goes back to the concept of 'body humours' by the Greeks. According to this theory, the melancholic was believed to have a predominance of 'black bile' mingling with his blood. Since those days, our ideas have changed, but the old name still persists.

6 Beneath the ribs At either side of the upper abdomen is a region designated the hypochondrium. Greek *hypo* is 'under' and *chondrium* implies' the cartilages of the ribs'. Discomfort here frequently provides the morbidly imaginative with ideas of disease, giving rise to the word hypochondriac – a person preoccupied with ill-health in spite of all reasonable reassurance to the contrary.

7 In yeast This word, derived from the Greek, means 'in yeast'. Human enzymes are the body's vital ferments. They regulate all aspects of our metabolism and without them our internal chemistry would come to an abrupt stop. The activity of yeast in the fermentation of alcohol led to the discovery of enzymes.

8 Anatomical bisexual Hermaphrodite is a combination of the names of Hermes (Mercury), the messenger of the Gods, and Aphrodite (Venus), Goddess of Beauty. Individuals are sometimes born in which the genitalia of females resemble those of males and vice-versa. Very rarely, true hermaphrodites are born who, in one body, possess the organs of reproduction of both sexes.

9 Half skull The classical symptom in migraine is a one-sided headache. This fact explains its name from a French corruption of the Greek *hemikrania* meaning 'half the skull'.The English 'megrim' is yet another variation. All refer to the condition colloquially known as 'bilious headache'.

10 A bunch of berries The Greek *staphyle* is 'a bunch of grapes' and coccus is 'a berry'. The staphylococci are a group of micro-organisms characterized by their growth in grape-like clusters. *Staphylococcus aureus,* found in the pus of infected wounds, is of prime clinical importance. Its ability to develop resistance to antibiotic drugs has become a matter of great concern.

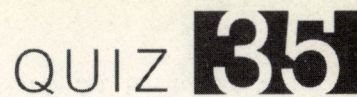

Which, what and why

When knowledge is limited – as is the case with medicine – it is always much easier to ask the questions than to supply the answers. Yet more knowledge means more queries and the process, like Swift's fleas, is a never ending one.

These questions here will test how well-informed you are on current medical knowledge.

1 Which arrow poison revolutionized anaesthesia?

2 What is cat gut?

3 Why do we pant after running for a bus?

4 Which disease is now recognized as 'top killer'?

5 What is thrush?

6 Why is it painful to bite on silver paper with a metallic tooth-filling?

7 What is myopia?

8 Which powerful brain stimulant was discovered in Mexican cacti?

9 What causes a wound to turn septic?

10 Why do we tan with sunshine?

answers overleaf

1 Curare Abdominal operations require profound muscular relaxation. This presented a major problem for the anaesthetist. It was achieved by deep unconsciousness – often approaching danger level. Curare was discovered as a South American arrow-poison which produced muscular paralysis. Its use in anaesthetics gives the required muscular relaxation at light and safe levels of anaesthesia.

2 Sheep's intestine 'Cat gut' is prepared from sheep's intestine. It is particularly useful for internal surgical stitches and obligingly disappears when the wounds have healed. Cat lovers can relax! – pussy's vitals play no part in the mysteries of surgical stitchcraft.

3 Oxygen debt For short, strenous outbursts of muscular activity, the body burns glucose much faster than oxygen can be supplied from the lungs for this purpose. In this way an 'oxygen debt' accumulates. The debt must later be paid off by over-breathing when the activity has finished. For this reason we continue to pant after taking our seat in the bus.

4 Heart disease Disease of the heart now ranks as top killer in most developed countries of the world. Can this be the price for civilization? Research into this illness is still incomplete and no one can at present say. Suspicion is thrown on the speed of modern life and the fats which are found in our diet. Men are more prone to the disease than women.

5 Fungal infection Thrush has nothing to do with the songbird. It is an infection by the vegetable fungus *Candida albicans*. It attacks mucous membranes and is typically found in the mouths of debilitated or poorly nourished children. It is seen as small white patches superficially resembling curdled milk.

6 Electrical phenomenon When silver paper comes into contact with a metallic tooth-filling, a simple electric cell is formed. Electricity flows from one metal to the other. This minute electric current stimulates the nerve of the tooth and sets up that sudden, unpleasant sensation of toothache, familiar to all who have eaten chocolate in a cinema.

7 Shortsightedness In this condition the eyeball is too long in shape and distant objects are therefore focussed to a point short of the light-sensitive retina. Concave spectacle lenses of appropriate strength correct the myopic error. The visual image will now fall exactly on the retina and the distant object will be clearly seen.

8 Mescaline This powerful drug – employed in modern psychiatric research – has already seen centuries of use at Mexican Indian religious ceremonies. It produces remarkable effects in the sense of sight. Illusions, dramatic visions and vivid colours are perceived in a setting of ecstasy. Mescaline belongs to the group of drugs known as 'phantastica'.

9 Bacteria A septic wound teems with bacteria. Multiplying in their millions, these germs fight to the death with the white cells of the blood. The resulting debris is called pus. Earlier medical ignorance welcomed pus formation as a necessary and laudable stage of healing. We now know that wounds heal best in the absence of infection of any kind.

10 Pigment formation Sunlight has a stimulating effect on the pigment cells found in the deepest layers of the skin. Chemical changes occur and increased amounts of the dark pigment melanin are produced. This pigment has primarily a protective function. Similar 'tanning' will occur at home with the aid of an ultraviolet lamp.

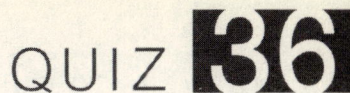

A quiz of quotes

Sickness and healing have pervaded the history of mankind like two forces of evil and good. Since earliest times, man's struggle with disease has fired the imagination of writers and poets. Small wonder that our literature abounds with medical references.

Here is a collection of better-known examples. How many of these can you identify?

1 Who was the fairies' midwife?

2 Who left his second leg (and the 42nd Foot) on the field of battle?

3 Who had medicine for breakfast, dinner and tea?

4 Who was cursed by infections of bogs, fens and flats?

5 Who was a very perfect practitioner?

6 Who was never, never sick at sea?

7 Who was from his mother's womb untimely ripped?

8 Who carried the bottle of medicine in her mouth?

9 Who declared 'We all labour against our own cure for death is the cure of all diseases.'

10 'Physicians of the utmost fame
Were called at once; but when they came
They answered, as they took their fees,
"There is no cure for this disease".'
But who was ill?

answers overleaf

1 **Queen Mab,** *Romeo and Juliet* Shakespeare gives a delightful account of this fairy – 'in shape no bigger than an agate-stone on the forefinger of an alderman'. Any unexplained mischief which occurred at night was readily attributed to her. As midwife, she delivered sleepers of their dreams, riding over them in her hazelnut chariot.

2 **Ben Battle,** *Faithless Nellie Gray* Soldier-hero of Hood's ballad, Ben lays down his arms on losing his legs. Arriving home, he finds the affections of his sweetheart Nelly displaced elsewhere – Some other man, Ben feels, is standing in his shoes. The blow is too great for our hero. Miss Gray's refusal to be his Nell proves to be the death of Ben.

3 **Tigger,** *The House at Pooh Corner* Tigger – with egotistic enthusiasm – found Roo's 'Strengthening Medicine' so pleasant he took it for breakfast, dinner and tea. It was in fact extract of malt. Piglet remained unimpressed. He confided to Pooh he felt Tigger had been strengthened quite enough.

4 **Caliban,** *The Tempest* Caliban's curse typifies the 'foul air' theory of disease so widely held in less enlightened times. The air itself was believed to be the cause of plague and pestilence and ingenious methods were used to cleanse and sweeten it. Physicians carried protective aromatic herbs, a practice which, interestingly enough, can still be seen today in the ceremonial nosegays of High Court Judges.

5 **Doctor of Physic,** *Canterbury Tales* Chaucer describes his Doctor of Physic as 'a verray parfit praktisour'. This medical man was, after the custom of his day, well-versed in the ancient medical works and was an expert astrologer. His diagnoses were made from his patients' horoscopes and their treatment effectively prescribed according to their stars!

6 **Captain Corcoran,** *H. M. S. Pinafore* This gallant naval commander affirmed that he was 'never, never sick at sea'. However, when pressed by his crew, he admitted an occasional lapse. Sea-sickness is not fully understood and may happen to the ablest of seamen. It is closely linked with a temporary disturbance of the ear's delicate balancing apparatus.

7 **Macduff,** *Macbeth* Mediaeval superstition set the greatest score by dramatic and unusual events which attended an infant's birth. Macbeth was killed by Macduff despite the Apparition's prophesy that 'none of woman born' could harm Macbeth. Macduff could lay claim to superior wizardry by virtue of his Caesarean birth.

8 **Nana,** *Peter Pan* Nana – children's nurse to the Darling family in Peter Pan – was a Newfoundland dog. Reasonably enough, she carried around the bottle of cough medicine in her mouth. Mr Darling, in a fit of ill-temper, chained her up in the yard. So began the children's flight to the Never-never Land and their adventures with Peter Pan.

9 **Sir Thomas Browne,** *Religio Medici* Both medical thought and English literature have been enriched by the writings of this eminent seventeenth-century doctor-philosopher. His greatest work *Religio Medici* examines the antagonistic views of Church and Medicine, so prevalent in his day. He practised at Norwich and received there a knighthood from Charles II.

10 **Henry King,** *Cautionary Tales* Hilaire Belloc warns of the plight of Henry King, reputedly cut off in Dreadful Agonies when internal knotting superceded his string-chewing habits. A likely story – and a less likely diagnosis! Why should Henry chew string in the first place? One is left with the uneasy suspicion that the whole issue could be explained by Henry's obsessive compulsion or perhaps hysteria.

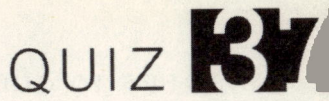
A change of name

The commercial naming of drugs is one of the plagues of modern medicine. A single chemical substance made by a dozen different manufacturers will masquerade under twelve different names – each with its own special claims to superior efficacy. The situation is ridiculous and openly fosters confusion.

Here, it is hoped, things are not quite so bad. Set out are ten medical substances, but each has a well-known, everyday name. What is the common name in each case?

1 Sodium sulphate

2 Nitrous oxide

3 Sucrose

4 Silver nitrate

5 Mercurous chloride

6 Ascorbic acid

7 Methyl salicylate

8 Hydrated calcium sulphate

9 Magnesium sulphate

10 Ammonium carbonate

answers overleaf

1 Glauber's salts Johann Glauber, the seventeenth century alchemist, made many interesting chemical discoveries. Among these was sodium sulphate, called by Glauber 'sal admirabile' but later known by the chemist's own name. It has a bitter taste and acts both as a laxative and diuretic. Glauber's salts are found naturally in the waters of many continental spas.

2 Laughing gas The anaesthetic effects of 'laughing gas' – earlier used in dental practice – were discovered by Sir Humphrey Davy in 1799. He, appropriately enough, was cutting a troublesome wisdom tooth at the time. His discovery met with little enthusiasm in England, where the gas was in keen demand for party frolics. Its far-reaching benefits to the field of anaesthetics were developed later in America.

3 Sugar Sucrose is normal household sugar. In spite of the important part it plays in our daily diet, sucrose cannot be absorbed by the body. It is broken down by the digestive juices to yield the simpler sugars of glucose and fructose. Cane sugar and beet sugar are of course identical substances and are merely other names for sucrose.

4 Lunar caustic This silver salt can be used for burning away warts and small unwanted tags of skin. Its properties were known to the alchemists of old and its history is an interesting one. Its name 'lunar caustic' still bears the mark of the ancient astrologers, who considered pale, gleaming silver to be the metal of the Moon.

5 Calomel Mercurous chloride is a white powder. Its alternative name of calomel means, oddly enough, 'beautiful black'. This paradox is explained by the striking change to a black powder which the salt undergoes if treated with ammonia. Medicinally, calomel may be used as a purgative.

6 Vitamin C Vitamin C prevents scurvy. In earlier times, this disease ravaged sailors confined for long voyages where fresh fruit and vegetables were unobtainable. The gums swelled and teeth dropped out. Wounds showed little tendency to heal.

Haemorrhages occurred throughout the body and frequently proved fatal. Generous quantities of ascorbic acid are found in lemons, oranges, blackcurrants and tomatoes.

7 Oil of wintergreen Oil of wintergreen is the methyl ester of salicylic acid, an acid closely related to aspirin. It has its own unmistakable smell and is a favourite component of liniments and antirheumatic ointments. Pharmacologically, it is classed as a counter-irritant. Its application to the skin relieves pain in underlying muscles, tendons and joints.

8 Plaster of Paris Surgery owes a special debt to this unassuming calcium compound. Originating from Montmartre in Paris, it revolutionized fracture healing and the treatment of orthopaedic deformities. When wet, it can be easily moulded to the individual needs of any patient. On setting, it provides full support for the injured part and effective immobilization of the damaged tissues.

9 Epsom salts These salts were named from their natural occurrence in the mineral springs at Epsom. When taken by mouth, they exert their purgative action by retaining water within the bowel and stimulating intestinal movement. A thick paste of magnesium sulphate makes a useful dressing in the treatment of boils and carbuncles.

10 Sal volatile This salt tends to disappear if left uncovered – hence its name of 'sal volatile'. It has been put to various uses in medicine and is frequently found as an ingredient of smelling salts. Taken internally, large doses of ammonium carbonate induce vomiting. Smaller doses can be very helpful for loosening a tight cough.

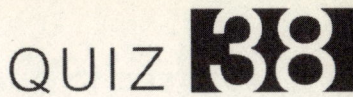

Medical Knowledge for Fun

Doctors' diseases

Many diseases, in addition to their formal medical titles, are sometimes known by a doctor's name. This doctor is usually found to have discovered the disease or to have supplied its original description.

Here are ten such diseases — each known by a doctor's name. Can you say what the illness is in each case?

1 Parkinson's disease

2 Bright's disease

3 Raynaud's disease

4 Hodgkin's disease

5 Pott's disease

6 Addison's disease

7 Buerger's disease

8 Weil's disease

9 Graves' disease

10 Ménière's disease

answers overleaf

1 Paralysis agitans James Parkinson described this illness in 1817. A peculiar trembling of the thumb and first finger is often the first sign to appear and gave the disease its old name of 'shaking palsy'. The muscles of the body show a slowly increasing stiffness. The disease most commonly occurs in elderly persons. Its cause lies in the central nervous system.

2 Nephritis Richard Bright, whose name became a byword for kidney disease, was a nineteenth century physician of Guy's Hospital. Until his time, little was understood in the condition of nephritis. Bright set out the fundamentals involved, correlating his clinical observations with the postmortem appearances of the diseased kidneys.

3 Spasm of digital arteries The hands of young women are particularly affected by Raynaud's disease. Paroxysmal attacks of arterial spasm cause the fingers to go white and dead. Cold is an important precipitating factor. Between attacks the fingers are quite normal. Maurice Raynaud practised in Paris and described the disease in 1882.

4 Lymphadenoma Hodgkin's disease affects the lymph glands. These show gross changes, enlarging painlessly and progressively. Eventually, a thick 'collar' of glands may surround the neck and the spleen is frequently involved. Through no fault of his own, Thomas Hodgkin's career was beset with disappointment. He eventually abandoned the practice of medicine.

5 Spinal tuberculosis The hunchback is a typical product of Pott's disease. The softened, tuberculous vertebrae are unable to take the weight imposed on them and collapse with angulation of the spine. Percival Pott was a colourful eighteenth century surgeon of St Bartholomew's Hospital. Pott's fracture-dislocation of the ankle is also named after him.

6 Adrenal insufficiency Muscular weakness, a low blood pressure and pigmentation of the skin are leading features of Addison's disease. Its cause is found in disease of the adrenal glands and is frequently tuberculous in origin. Thomas Addison was a famous physician and clinical teacher at Guy's Hospital. He was the first to discover and describe pernicious anaemia.

7 Thromboangiitis obliterans Buerger's disease attacks the blood vessels of the legs. Thrombosis occurs and scar tissue formation follows. The blood flow to the muscles is severely reduced and acute pain in the calves is commonly experienced after walking short distances. The pain passes on resting a while. King George VI suffered from this condition.

8 Haemorrhagic jaundice Minute wriggling microbes, found in the urine of rats, are the causal agents of this disease. Outbreaks occur where rats are plentiful, and incidence is high among sewer workers, coal miners and farm workers. Fever, jaundice and haemorrhages are leading symptoms. Adolf Weil described the condition in 1886.

9 Exophthalmic goitre This condition represents a classical form of thyrotoxicosis, with typical protruding eyes and a swollen thyroid gland in the neck. Women are affected far more frequently than men. Robert Graves was physician to the Meath Hospital, Dublin. Although not the first to describe this condition, his name has designated it for over a hundred years.

10 Aural vertigo Excess fluid within the balancing apparatus of the ear is held to be the cause of this disorder. Its attacks can be sudden and dramatic. The patient frequently senses that everything is spinning round and may fall to the floor and vomit. Prosper Ménière, Director of the Institution for Deaf Mutes in Paris, described the condition in his last year of life.

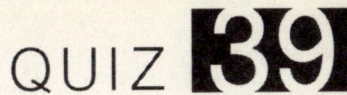
Quaint and curious

Certain medical conditions are well known by their everyday names. These are often very descriptive and not infrequently colourful.

Here is a quiz of the quaint and curious. Can you say what these really are?

1 Cauliflower ear

2 Saturday night paralysis

3 Moon face

4 Derbyshire neck

5 Hobnail liver

6 Tennis elbow

7 Cheshire cat smile

8 Horseshoe kidney

9 Harelip

10 Athlete's foot

answers overleaf

1 Fibrosis of the ear This is the condition of the prize-fighter. Repeated blows on the outer ear cause multiple bleeding into its tissues. The resulting blood clots are slowly replaced by fibrous tissue which then undergoes contraction. The contraction grossly distorts the outer ear, gathering the flesh into the characteristic, puckered, cauliflower-like folds.

2 Radial nerve palsy The radial nerve winds around the back of the upper arm close to the bone. Prolonged compression of this nerve will give rise to a temporary paralysis of those muscles which bend back the wrist and arm. A drunken sleep with the arms dangling over the side of a chair was at one time a frequent cause. Hence its name, 'Saturday night paralysis'.

3 Hydration of the face A face like a harvest moon – large, fat, round and shining – sometimes occurs in a patient receiving certain medicines. Cortisone is a prime example. The cause is that of fluid retention within the tissues of the face. With discontinuation of the drug, the 'moon face' wanes and soon resumes more earthly proportions.

4 Simple goitre The soil of Derbyshire is poor in iodine – an element essential for normal function of the thyroid gland. Starved of iodine, the frustrated thyroid gland enlarges and may attain considerable size. Outwardly, the enlarged gland is seen as a 'goitre', conspicuous at the front of the neck and at one time endemic among Derbyshire patients.

5 Hepatic cirrhosis Excessive and chronic consumption of alcohol predisposes to cirrhosis of the liver. The normal cells of this organ are replaced by scar tissue and the liver becomes a shrunken fibrous mass. Small 'hobnails' of surviving liver tissue are squeezed out from the surface and lend the appearance of the studded undersurface of an old army boot.

6 Muscle strain Torn muscle fibres at the outermost point of the elbow are most commonly responsible for the pain of 'tennis elbow'. Occasionally, a ruptured ligament may contribute. Tennis players can claim no monopoly of this condition. It occurs in manual labourers and in enthusiastic violinists.

7 Facial myotonia Certain rare muscular disorders are characterized by an inability of the muscles to relax normally after contracting. One striking example of this will sometimes be seen in the patient's face. After smiling, the smile persists and then fades only gradually from the expression. This effect received its name from Lewis Carroll's enigmatic Cheshire Cat.

8 Conjoined kidneys On certain occasions, the two kidneys fail to develop separately and remain joined at their lower ends. From its appearance, this single organ is termed a 'horseshoe kidney'. As such, it can be quite consistent with a normal healthy life and need give rise to no symptoms whatsoever.

9 Malformation of the upper lip The human face develops in three distinct parts. Defective union of these components is commonly seen as a 'harelip' – sometimes accompanied by a cleft palate. The fissure in the upper lip lies just to one side of the midline. More rarely, it may be present on both sides. Fortunately, the 'harelip' is completely remediable by plastic surgery.

10 Fungal infection This condition is caused by a parasitic mould. Such fungi belong to the plant kingdom but having no green chlorophyll cannot make glucose. Thus, they obtain their nutrient from organic material – in this case the skin. The disease is caught from infected clothes, socks, towels and damp mats.

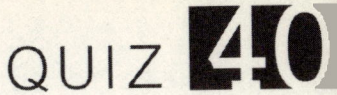

Medical Knowledge for Fun

Great saints

Prolonged suffering formed the traditional setting for the ancient saintly life – but times have presumably changed. Today, most of us are reaching for the crown of martyrdom after only three days with a heavy head cold. The pace of modern living obviously speeds things up.

Certain saints have their special associations with medicine and here are ten examples. Solve each clue and name each saint.

1 Master of the Dance.

2 Surgical twins – Arabian not Siamese.

3 Saint with the blues from a very bad headache.

4 He sounds doubtful but isn't.

5 The blacksmith who cares for the blind.

6 The doctor–disciple.

7 An incendiary prebendary?

8 The crusader bears his cross.

9 The serenade of the gondolier.

10 Small baron in the city.

answers overleaf

1 St Vitus St Vitus, patron saint of dancers and actors, was martyred by being cast into a cauldron of boiling oil. During the seventeenth century, a belief was prevalent that good health could be secured for the coming year by dancing before the saint's image at his annual festival. His compassion was sought for rheumatic chorea – a disease later known as St Vitus' dance.

2 St Cosmas and St Damian These saints were twin brothers who together wrought many surgical miracles. They were Arabian by birth and devoted their lives to the study of medicine and healing the sick. In the course of their persecution, they survived drowning, burning and stoning but were eventually beheaded. St Cosmas and St Damian became the patron saints of surgery.

3 St Louis This saint's name has passed to medicine via the Missouri town named after him in the United States. In 1933, hundreds of its occupants were smitten with an inflammation of the brain, caused by a hitherto unknown virus. Since that time, further cases have occurred each year in America and the condition is known as St Louis encephalitis.

4 St Thomas à Becket St Thomas à Becket was murdered in Canterbury cathedral. To this saint was originally dedicated St Thomas's Hospital in 1215. Some three hundred years later, King Henry VIII declared the saint a traitor and caused the destruction of his shrine and the re-dedication of the hospital to St Thomas the Apostle. Florence Nightingale established her famous first nursing school at St Thomas's Hospital.

5 St Dunstan St Dunstan's organization exists for the care and rehabilitation of men and women blinded on war service. St Dunstan himself was a blacksmith and something of a character. On one occasion, according to legend, he seized the devil by the nose with his red-hot tongs. St Dunstan became Abbot of Glastonbury and later was made Archbishop of Canterbury.

6 St Luke St Luke, devoted companion to St Paul, was a physician by profession. Little is known about his life and med-

ical practice. Traditionally, he is believed also to have been an artist and is the patron saint of painters. It is St Paul in the *Epistle to the Colossians* who describes him as 'Luke, the beloved physician'.

7 St Anthony Epidemics of 'St Anthony's fire' have plagued mankind at intervals throughout the ages. This condition is ergot poisoning, acquired from eating diseased rye – though the same name has sometimes been used for the infection of erysipelas. St Anthony was an Egyptian abbot and is usually remembered for his many temptations.

8 St John At the time of the first crusade, the urgent need for medical and nursing services was met by the newly formed Order of St John. Its Knights Hospitaller tended the sick in their own hospital at Jerusalem. With the fall of Jerusalem, the Knights sought refuge at Rhodes and later removed to Malta. The Maltese Cross is still found in the uniform of St John's Ambulance Brigade.

9 St Lucia St Lucia, born at Syracuse, is patron saint of eyes and their diseases. To discourage one pagan suitor, so legend affirms, she plucked out her own eyes and sent them to him in a dish. The remorse-stricken pagan became a Christian and St Lucia's sight was miraculously restored.

10 St Bartholomew St Bartholomew the Apostle gives his name to the oldest of London's hospitals. 'Barts' was founded in 1123 at Smithfield by Rahere, an Augustinian Canon. Earlier, this monk had been desperately ill in Rome and, on returning to England, established the hospital in gratitude for deliverance from death. Rahere, at one time, was jester to the Court of Henry I.

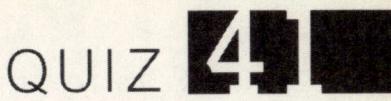
Medical Knowledge for Fun

Doctor in disguise

Ten doctors, drawn from life and literature, provide the answers to this quiz. Side-by-side, they form an incongruous group yet each as an individual achieved public renown.

Solve the clues and find the physicians!

1 Signatory to the devil.

2 'Elementary, my dear...'

3 Father to the world's largest family.

4 Hispaniola's surgeon.

5 W. G.

6 Philosopher-musician-theologian-physician.

7 The missing wire tripped him and caught him.

8 His own better half.

9 Presumptive discovery proved perfectly right.

10 The monster maker.

answers overleaf

1 Faust As far as we can tell, a notorious Dr Faust actually existed in Germany during the early sixteenth century. He travelled the country swindling and cheating with fake-healing and necromancy. His violent and unexplained death was readily put down to the work of the devil. This theme inspired the magnificent tragedies of Marlowe and Goethe.

2 Watson Dr John Watson shared lodgings with Sherlock Holmes at 221B Baker Street, London. His good-humoured naivety and ponderous thinking formed the perfect foil for Holmes' deductive brilliance. Their creator, Sir Arthur Conan Doyle, was himself a medical man and is believed to have modelled Holmes on his old clinical teacher – the famous Dr Joseph Bell of Edinburgh.

3 Barnardo Dr Thomas Barnardo was born in Dublin in 1845. He studied medicine at the London Hospital intending to become a medical missionary, but then opened his home for destitute children at Stepney in East London. Since that time, his organization has cared for hundreds of thousands of children. No child in need has ever been refused.

4 Livesey Dr Livesey was the country practitioner in Stevenson's *Treasure Island*. He sailed as ship's doctor on the *Hispaniola* with his friends Jim Hawkins and Squire Trelawney in search of the pirate treasure. Livesey's sound judgement befitting a medical man offset the irresponsibilities of Trelawney and played a major part in the overthrow of the pirates and the successful conclusion of the adventure.

5 Grace Dr W.G. Grace was the greatest of all cricketers. His now-legendary figure stood over six feet at the wicket and was surmounted with a striking black beard. Although medically qualified, Dr Grace devoted his life to the game at which he excelled. Captain of Gloucester and captain of England, he scored over 54 000 runs in first-class cricket.

6 Schweitzer Having already graduated in philosophy, in theology and in music, Dr Albert Schweitzer realized his true life's work lay as a medical missionary. He then studied and qualified in medicine, prior to building his own missionary hospital at Lambarene in Africa. The human approach and practical help of this incredible man have relieved the suffering of thousands. The world acknowledged its debt to Dr Schweitzer and awarded him, among many other honours, the Nobel Peace Prize.

7 Crippen The infamous Dr Crippen murdered his wife with hyoscine. After dissecting her body, he buried the remains in his cellar and made off for America, accompanied by his mistress who had disguised herself as a boy. Crippen made history as the first criminal to be arrested at sea on information passed by the recently introduced wireless.

8 Jekyll In Stevenson's well-known story, Dr Jekyll experiments upon himself with his newly prepared drugs and stumbles upon the means of completely transforming himself. By day he remains the doctor, but by night changes to the depraved criminal – Mr Hyde. At first, he is able to control and reverse these changes but later this power is lost. In desperation, he takes his own life.

9 Livingstone Dr David Livingstone, the indomitable explorer of Central Africa, qualified at Glasgow in 1840. He sailed for Bechuanaland as a medical missionary, but in 1849 set forth on his famous travels. He explored the Zambesi, discovered Victoria Falls and found many of the great African lakes. He died of dysentery on an expedition to trace the source of the Nile. His body was brought to England and is buried in Westminster Abbey.

10 Frankenstein Mary Shelley, wife of the poet Percy Bysshe Shelley, wrote her famous story of *Frankenstein* in 1818. In it, the spine-chilling Dr Frankenstein creates a monster from spare body parts purloined from graves and then brings his creation to life. So often the name Frankenstein is wrongly applied to the monster itself when in fact it was the name of the bizarre doctor who created it.

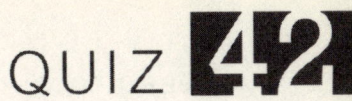
Human geometry

No advanced knowledge of Euclid or Pythagoras is required for this quiz. Many named geometrical entities can be found in the human body. Each serves a specific role in function or diagnosis.

Can you name where the following are located?

1 The radius

2 The pyramids

3 The trapezius

4 McBurney's point

5 The angle of Louis

6 The triangle of auscultation

7 The cerebral hemispheres

8 The semicircular canals

9 The apex beat

10 The circle of Willis

answers overleaf

1 The arm The radius is one of two bones found in the fore-arm and is named from its resemblance to the spoke of a wheel. Its widened, lower end articulates with the wrist bones and indirectly carries the hand. The important twisting movements of the hand – as when using a screwdriver – are produced by rotations of the radius.

2 The brain The pyramids are found on the surface of the medulla oblongata – that portion of the brain which is continuous with the spinal cord. They are seen as two eminences and are raised by the nerve fibres which stream down from the brain into the spinal cord to control the voluntary muscular movements of the body.

3 The back The trapezius muscle lies in the upper part of the back, positioned rather like a monk's cowl. It is attached to the skull above, to the shoulder blade of each side and to the dorsal vertebrae of the spinal column. Its principle actions are seen in shrugging the shoulders and in maintaining a good posture with the shoulders well back.

4 The abdomen At the upper and outermost part of the groin a bony prominence of the hip bone can be felt. McBurney's point lies about an inch-and-a-half along a line drawn from here to the navel. This point indicates the classical site of maximum tenderness in acute appendicitis and is the surgeon's landmark when operating for this condition.

5 The chest On the front of the chest, some two inches from the top of the sternum or breast bone, a rough, transverse, bony ridge can be felt with the fingers. This is the 'angle of Louis', formed by the attachment of the 'handle' to the 'blade' of the sternum. This angle provides the starting point for counting the ribs and marks the attachment of the second rib.

6 The back A small triangular area can be found near the lowest point of the shoulder blade, where the thick muscular coverings of the back are absent. A stethoscope applied here will pick up the sounds of the chest particularly well. This area is accordingly named the triangle of 'auscultation' – the technical term for 'listening-in'.

7 The brain Our cerebrum – the greatest portion of our brain – is divided longitudinally into two well-marked hemispheres. Each hemisphere controls the opposite side of the body. In right-handed persons, the left hemisphere is 'dominant' and will contain the speech centre of the brain. In left-handed persons, this situation is reversed.

8 The ear The labyrinth of the inner ear, set deep within the bone of the skull, contains three semicircular canals. These have nothing to do with hearing but are organs of balance. They are arranged at right angles to each other and are filled with fluid. Movements of this fluid inform us of the movements of our head in space.

9 The chest The apex beat is felt and sometimes seen on the left side of the chest. It is the thrust of the contracting heart against the chest wall. Its position is a guide in assessing enlargement of the heart. The apex beat is usually found in the fifth rib-space, some three to four inches from the midline of the chest.

10 The brain Thomas Willis described this 'circle' of arteries found at the base of the brain surrounding the pituitary gland. Willis was Professor of Natural Philosophy at Oxford in the time of Charles II and published a classical work on the anatomy of the brain in 1664. Illustrations for this were drawn by his versatile and gifted pupil – the famous Christopher Wren.

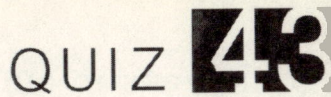

Medical Knowledge for Fun

Do-it-yourself diagnosis

A quick glance at a television screen, some urgent thumbing of a medical dictionary, and many individuals already see themselves as heaven's gift to medical diagnosis. The procedure is an unwise one and can be very dangerous. For all that, certain clear cut symptoms can suggest certain diseases. You are invited here to consider the likely diagnosis in each of the following cases.

1 The bones of an undernourished and sun-starved child have bent with the weight of their body.

2 Uncontrolled bleeding is found in the male members of a certain family.

3 Difficulty in seeing is found to be due to an increasing opacity of the lens of the eye.

4 A patient who complains of pain in the great toe is found to have chalky lumps in the ear.

5 A person recently returned from the tropics complains of bouts of high temperature with shivering which occur at regular intervals.

6 Sugar is found in the urine of a patient who experiences excessive thirst.

7 Spasm of the jaw muscles follows an unclean flesh wound.

8 An elderly person is suddenly struck with a paralysis down the whole of one side of the body.

9 A most painful area of hard skin on a toe.

10 A gentleman in his fifties finds he must hold a newspaper further and further away to read it clearly.

answers overleaf

1 Rickets Rickets is caused by deficiency of vitamin D – an essential for healthy bone formation. Without this vitamin, the bones of a growing child bend beneath the weight of the body, producing deformed and twisted limbs. Vitamin D is plentiful in fish liver oils. It can be synthesized by the action of sunlight on the skin.

2 Haemophilia This disease runs in families. It occurs in the males but is passed to succeeding generations by the females. The blood is unable to clot normally and severe haemorrhages may follow trivial injuries. Tooth extractions require special precautions. Advanced treatment is now available for haemophiliacs.

3 Cataract The causes of cataract are many. This condition can run in families, may follow injury or an illness such as diabetes, or equally may be just one feature of growing old. Fortunately, a relatively simple operation can restore the sight in many cases, whereby a tiny plastic lens is fitted in place of the normal lens of the eye.

4 Gout A popular but mistaken belief attributed gout to over-indulgence in the better things of life. It is in fact a disorder of the body's chemistry. Abnormal amounts of uric acid circulate in the blood and deposits of urate crystals appear in the tissues. A favourite site is the joints of the big toe. Hereditary factors play a large part in the incidence of this disease.

5 Malaria Attacks of high fever, with regular recurrence at intervals of two or three days, suggest malaria in those who have served abroad. Malaria parasites, injected by the bite of an infected mosquito, multiply in the red corpuscles and periodically burst in their thousands into the bloodstream. At these times, the temperature soars and the typical bouts of uncontrollable shaking are seen.

6 Diabetes Those suffering from 'sugar diabetes' cannot utilize glucose properly. This fault is due to lack of insulin – the internal secretion of the pancreas gland. Excessive quantities of sugar accumulate in the blood and in the tissues. The kidney attempts to reduce these amounts by excreting glucose into the urine.

7 Tetanus Tetanus, otherwise known as 'lockjaw', is caused by a bacterium which abounds in well-manured soils. Its poison attacks the central nervous system, giving rise to the muscular spasms which characterize this disease. Soil-contaminated wounds should never be neglected. The treatment of such wounds may require a protective injection of antitetanus serum.

8 Stroke A stroke is caused by a central haemorrhage or clot (thrombus) forming *in situ* within the brain. Alternatively, it may be by an 'infarct' – a particle of detritus in the cardiovascular system which is trundled along to the brain until it meets an artery too small for it when it acts as a plug cutting off the blood supply. Since the nerve fibres cross over, the site of cerebral damage will lie on the opposite side of the brain to the paralysed side of the body.

9 Corn There is nothing surprising about the formation of a corn. This small plug of intensely hardened skin forms to protect the foot from localized pressure or friction from an ill-fitting shoe. The corn itself is quite insensitive but once formed transfers any further pressure directly onto the sensitive nerve endings lying beneath. Result: exquisite agony!

10 Presbyopia This is 'old sight'. In middle age and subsequently the lens of the eye loses its elasticity and cannot obtain its convexity of earlier years. In consequence, the near point of vision recedes and objects must be held further and further away to bring them into focus. Glasses with biconvex lenses can correct this condition.

Medical Knowledge for Fun

Madam and medicine

Since the Garden of Eden, woman's influence in human affairs has been all-embracing. The hand that rocks the cradle is equally capable of rocking the boat – and, in this case, the backwash may well sink a battleship or, like Helen of Troy, launch a thousand ships.

    For what in the healing arts are the following women renowned?

1 Medea

2 'James' Barry

3 Lady Mary Montagu

4 Elizabeth Blackwell

5 Marie Curie

6 Elizabeth Kenny

7 Florence Nightingale

8 Mary Donally

9 Countess of Chinchon

10 Edith Louisa Cavell

answers overleaf

1 Transfusion In Greek mythology, Medea was Queen of Colchis and wife of Jason, seeker of the Golden Fleece. She doctored by the darker arts and excelled with her fantastic potions and herbal brews. Her enchanted transfusion of Jason's aged father completely rejuvenated the old man and foreshadowed the events of centuries to come. Today, however, Medea's principles would have had her stuck from any medical register.

2 A pseudo-male This enigmatic doctor joined the British Army as a male surgeon in 1813. For years, Barry gave distinguished medical service in many parts of the world and eventually was rewarded with the high-ranking appointment of Inspector General of Hospitals. At death, an extraordinary discovery was made. This foremost military surgeon was found to be a woman!

3 Smallpox inoculation In the early eighteenth century, Lady Mary Wortley Montagu, wife of the English ambassador at Constantinople, first introduced into England a method of inoculation against smallpox. This was the Eastern practice of direct inoculation from patient to patient. The method was not without its dangers and later gave place to the safe technique of vaccination.

4 First woman medical graduate Elizabeth Blackwell claims pride of place as the first qualified woman doctor. Until the mid-nineteenth century, medicine was jealously guarded as the strict province of the male. Born in England, Miss Blackwell studied in America and qualified in New York in 1849. Her reluctant acceptance by the profession marked a radical and far-reaching victory over current medical prejudice.

5 Discovery of radium Marie Curie was twice awarded a Nobel Prize. After studying at the Sorbonne and obtaining the highest distinctions of that University, she began work with her husband on the analysis of pitchblende. Their combined efforts led to their discovery and isolation of radium. The use of radium in the treatment of cancer became later known as 'Curie-therapy'.

6 Revolution of polio treatment This Australian Nursing Sister revolutionized the management of poliomyelitis. Against bitter medical opposition she denounced the practice of splinting the paralysed limbs or encasing them in plaster. The muscles, she insisted, required heat, bathing and exercises to relax their spasms. Her principles are now universally accepted. President Roosevelt, himself a polio victim, welcomed her to America.

7 Lady of the lamp In 1854, the Barrack Hospital at Scutari reeked with its filth, squalor and infestation. Here the British wounded from the Crimea lay dying from neglect. Here too, bristling with compassion and efficiency, came Florence Nightingale having overcome considerable political opposition. Result: transformation of that terrible scene and the establishment of the principles of modern nursing. Miss Nightingale – the lady of the lamp – was awarded the Order of Merit in 1907.

8 First live Caesarean birth Although live children had been delivered from dying mothers since ancient times, it was Mary Donally, an unqualified midwife, who performed the first successful Caesarean operation in Britain, whereby both mother and child lived. The mother had been in labour for ten days. Mary Donally delivered her child to the living mother in 1738.

9 Countess's powder According to legend, the Countess of Chinchon, seventeenth century wife of the Viceroy of Peru, lay desperately ill with fever. She was dramatically saved by a powder prepared from tree bark. This then became famous as 'Countess' powder'. It was in fact an early preparation of quinine.

10 National heroine During World War I, Nurse Edith Louisa Cavell continued as Matron of the École Belge d'Infirmières Diplomées in Brussels. On August 5th 1915, she was arrested by the Germans, charged with harbouring refugees and helping them to escape. She was tried, sentenced to death and shot. A wave of horror swept the world. Her body was brought to England and buried in Norwich Cathedral.

Food – fact or fad

Food, for most of us, is more than a bare necessity of life. To many, it has become an ingrained and trendy attitude of mind. The dream of the epicure is the nightmare of the faddist; the trencherman's delight is the hypochondriac's bane.

Where food is concerned, fact and fad are often hopelessly mixed. Here is a selection of both. Can you sort out which is which among the examples given here?

1 Brown eggs are more nutritious than white.

2 Christmas disease is caused by seasonal overeating.

3 Potatoes are fattening.

4 Drinking hot tea will cool one.

5 We each require a pint of milk per day.

6 Asparagus is unwholesome.

7 We each shall eat a peck of dirt before we die.

8 Duck eggs are safer boiled than fried.

9 Red meat juice is specially good for the blood.

10 Eating beetroot colours the urine.

answers overleaf

1 Fad There is no truth in this widely held fallacy. The egg is a highly concentrated food store designed by nature for the developing chick embryo. Its yolk contains a mixture of fats and its white is the protein albumin. Brown eggs may look more attractive than white but have no superior nutritive value.

2 Fad Christmas disease has nothing to do with the seasonal festivities of December. It is a rare disorder of the blood closely allied to haemophilia. The fault lies in the blood's clotting and simple injuries are liable to cause serious bleeding. This disease was recognized in 1952 and is named after Stephen Christmas, the first patient.

3 Fact Like other starchy foods, potatoes consist mainly of carbohydrate. Carbohydrates are broken down to simple sugars during digestion and after absorption provide our principal source of physical energy. Quantities surplus to energy requirements are built up into fats and are stored away as such in the body's reserve depots.

4 Fad Drinking hot tea invariably makes us hotter. As we later resume our previous temperature, we may perhaps feel 'cooler' by comparison. The logic of this practice has much in common with that of hitting oneself on the head with a hammer – 'because it is so nice when one stops'.

5 Fad Milk is an excellent food. It is rich in protein, fat and carbohydrate and contains beneficial mineral salts and vitamins. For all this, milk is by no means an essential food. When adequate supplies of nutrition are obtained from other sources, we can live quite happily and quite healthily without it.

6 Fad Believe this and you will miss one of life's great delicacies. Asparagus with butter is not only delicious but can make a beneficial and satisfying meal. The fear of 'unwholesomeness' doubtless springs from the fact that, in certain people, eating asparagus imparts a harmless yet very disagreeable odour to the urine.

7 Fad Whatever truth this saying might – or might not – have had in the bad old days, modern standards of hygiene leave no justification for assuming we are doomed to eat two gallons (one peck) of dirt before we die. Certain children – and even some adults – may pass through phases of dirt-eating but these special cases fall outside the scope of this oft quoted proverb.

8 Fact Duck eggs may harbour salmonella germs – bacteria well-known for causing food poisoning. These germs can be killed by heat. For this reason duck eggs should always be very well cooked. Quick frying should be avoided – this can heat the outside of the egg yet leave the inside unaffected. Boiling for several minutes is very much safer.

9 Fad Red juice from underdone meat plays no special part in building human blood. Similarity of appearance may too easily lead us to associate this juice with our blood but the concept is too simple and discounts those changes the meat juice undergoes during digestion. Meat and its juices are highly nutritious and an excellent source of animal protein.

10 Fact Many a lover of beetroot, anxiously clutching a specimen of red urine, has consulted the doctor for 'blood in the water'. This condition, lightheartedly known as 'beeturia', fortunately requires only a little reassurance. The pigment of beetroot is excreted by the kidney and colours the urine red.

Find the fever

Fevers have routed armies, decimated nations and broken empires. Throughout the ages, man's dread of fevers seems only to have been exceeded by his dread of treatment, the standard version of which for any fever was 'starving, purgation and bleeding'.

Nowadays, most fevers respond to the gentler treatment of antibiotics. They have many forms and many facets. Here are ten which vary widely. Solve each clue and find each fever.

1 Spring breeze brings sneeze.

2 Caused by the cure.

3 Labour's unjust reward?

4 Those craves for the waves.

5 Earlier pestilence of prisons.

6 Sanitation into drinking water equals...

7 Amorous adolescent with a large neck.

8 This red would be found in bed.

9 This illness licks the joints and bites the heart.

10 Fever from a George Cross-island.

answers overleaf

1 Hay fever This is an allergic reaction normally occuring in spring or early summer. Sensitivity to pollens, from trees, grasses and plants causes great distress with sneezing, watering of the eyes and headache. Antihistamines, steroids and preparations of adrenalin all are found to relieve the condition in specific cases.

2 Drug fever Certain patients show an idiosyncrasy to some medicines and may react to these with fever. Penicillin and the sulphonamides have become well known for producing this effect. Other symptoms may appear and vary from a mild skin rash to those of a state of acute collapse. Anyone with a known drug sensitivity must always make this known to any practitioner who may treat them.

3 Puerperal fever In earlier times, this streptococcal infection was feared by all mothers newly delivered of their infants. Maternity wards were hotbeds of infection since the germs were unwittingly transferred from patient to patient on the hands of the midwives. Death rates were appalling. In 1847 at Vienna, Ignaz Semmelweiss demonstrated the dramatic reduction of deaths by the simple precaution of handwashing.

4 Sea fever Inasmuch as this has any specific medical meaning, it falls into the psychological category of 'overvalued idea'. This term denotes ideas which are born of very strong feelings. They may direct and dominate a person's whole life. They are frequently met as illogical cravings, fanatical enthusiasms or the irrepressible 'bee in the bonnet'.

5 Typhus fever Typhus is spread by the body louse. Outbreaks occur where standards of personal hygiene reach their lowest levels. It flourished among the dreadful conditions found in prisons of earlier centuries and earned for itself the name of 'gaol fever'. During World War II, typhus claimed hundreds of victims in the notorious concentration camp of Belsen.

6 Typhoid fever The spread of typhoid depends on a stark and unpleasant fact. A portion of some person's infected excreta finds its way into another person's mouth. Flies are the principal intermediaries in this unpalatable transmission and should be ruthlessly destroyed. 'Typhoid carriers' are persons who harbour the germs yet themselves show no outward signs of the disease.

7 Glandular fever This disease has proved something of an enigma. Its causative agent appears to be that of a virus and it primarily affects children and adolscents. Epidemics may occur and kissing has been blamed as one mode of transmission. The glands of the neck are principally involved and jaundice may occur in some patients.

8 Scarlet fever This fever is caused by the streptococcus – a chain-like bacterium with an 'erythrogenic' or red-producing toxin which causes the characteristic rash. Its occurence is most frequently in children of about five years old. It was prone to occur in epidemics and in earlier centuries had a very high mortality rate. Fortunately, the whole threat and incidence of scarlet fever has been changed by modern antibiotics.

9 Rheumatic fever This fever is caused by a streptococcal bacterium and in earlier times was a widespread problem in children. Its symptoms vary in that severity and mild attacks on the joints were often put down to 'growing pains'. The illness has a specific tendency to affect the heart, resulting in cardiac damage.

10 Malta fever This fever recurs and is known as undulant. It arises particularly in goat-rearing districts of the tropics and sub-tropics. Its symptoms are sweating, pains in the muscles, arthritis and an enlarged spleen caused by bacterial infection. Its occurrence in Malta gives its name to the disease.

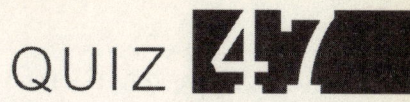
Which doctor

From medical man to medicine man, there is no doubt that doctors differ. Specialization involves differentiation and their work often varies as widely as themselves.

Here are a selection of specialities in medicine. Can you name the doctor who practises in each?

1 Mental disorders

2 Children's diseases

3 Painlessness

4 Diseases of women

5 Skin diseases

6 Postmortem examinations

7 Organic nervous diseases

8 Diseases of the aged

9 X-ray photography

10 Childbirth

95

answers overleaf

1 Psychiatrist The psychiatrist is a physician who has specialized in mental illness. He should not be confused with the psychologist who is rarely medically qualified nor the psychoanalyst who practises the strict analytical doctrines of Freud. Inestimable relief is at last being brought to mental suffering by the informed outlook of modern psychiatrists and their scientific use of the psychotropic medicines available.

2 Paediatrician Children – we are told – say the most peculiar things. They certainly get the most peculiar things wrong with them. Newly exposed to the germs of this world, they have yet to attain full natural immunity. Their response to infection is perplexing and individual. Examining them is an art in itself. This is well seen in the paediatrician – the children's own specialist.

3 Anaesthetist This doctor – sometimes affectionately known as the 'gasman' – applies the science of insensibility. At operations, he is found at the head of the table controlling the patient's degree of unconsciousness to the surgeon's activities. Without him, modern surgery would be impossible. In all medicine, no one does more for the relief of pain than the anaesthetist.

4 Gynaecologist This highly skilled surgeon treats the disorders of the female reproductive system. These disorders have their origins in many fields of medicine and surgery. The activities of the gynaecologist range widely – from treating glandular disturbances with hormones to the safe delivery of an infant by Caesarean operation.

5 Dermatologist Skin diseases are readily seen. Their dramatic appearances cause much unnecessary alarm. The dermatologist includes full use of reassurance when treating his patient and is familiar of the extent to which psychological factors can play their part in the causation of skin diseases. The skin has been called 'the mirror of the mind'.

6 Pathologist In the laboratory and postmortem room, the pathologist constantly seeks information to aid the clinician in his diagnoses and treatment. His investigations include blood tests, assessments of the body's chemistry, the identification of infecting germs and the examination of diseased tissues. Pathology is the fundamental science of medicine.

7 Neurologist The neurologist deals with organic disease occurring in the brain, spinal cord or peripheral nerves. His examination tests the 'circuits' of the nervous system – rather as one might test the wiring of an intricate electrical instrument. These healthy nervous circuits are essential for normal sensation and muscular movement. They provide the basis for all reflex actions.

8 Geriatrician Prolonging life with the 'wonder drugs' of today has in turn created its own problem for medical science. How best can the old folk be cared for and treated? Their specialized needs are the concern of the geriatrician, who is spending much time and thought in research in this field. The aged of yesterday have become the middle-aged of today.

9 Radiologist The use of X-rays – their role in treatment and the examination and interpretation of their photographic plates – calls for an expert with a highly technical training. This is the radiologist, the doctor who has specialized in this important branch of medicine. X-ray photography affords one of the greatest aids to diagnosis we possess.

10 Obstetrician The 'ordeal of childbirth' is now as dead as the dodo. The skill of the obstetrician has replaced it with a modern, safe and relatively painless technique. Much of its secret lies in efficient antenatal supervision and care. Early prevention of hazards is the secret of smooth and successful confinements.

Mixed bag

Here is a set of medical anagrams.

Rearrange the capital letters of each to form an item commonly found in a doctor's bag. Help can be found in the accompanying clues and the figures in brackets denote the number of letters in each word or words required for the answer.

1 REMOTER THEM – but the personal touch is quite essential *(11)*

2 NIP – ow! *(3)*

3 PERUSE A MAT – and discover its dimensions *(4,7)*

4 GANGLING MISS FAY – observed much larger than life *(10,5)*

5 AM REAL METAL HARP – and, am, of course, ready for many hard knocks *(8,6)*

6 TRICEL CROCHET – for something light and bright *(8,5)*

7 CORPSE F – pinched but not stolen *(7)*

8 YE MODERN PHYSIC RIG – but one still gets the old-fashioned point *(10,7)*

9 H SPY GAME OR MOMENT – resistance encircled under pressure *(16)*

10 POSE THE COST – then listen for the rumpus *(11)*

answers overleaf

1 Thermometer The clinical thermometer is simple yet ingenious. Just above its mercury bulb is found a small constriction. This ensures the maximum body temperature will remain recorded on the scale until the mercury column is forcibly shaken down once again. A small piece of the thermometer's wall magnifies and allows the temperature to be easily read.

2 Pin Our objection to jabs from the business end of a pin speaks well for the healthy state of our nervous system. So too does our ability, when our eyes are shut, to know if the sharp or blunt end is being used. Such sensory discrimination demands a high degree of nervous efficiency. The pin is an effective medical instrument.

3 Tape measure Doctors – like film stars – find physical measurements a great aid to successful treatment. Medical measuring graces itself with the high-sounding name of 'mensuration'. The tape measure has helped solve many a medical problem – from the diagnosis of twins to the demonstration of a broken limb.

4 Magnifying glass The magnifying glass is most useful for dealing with minor troubles of the skin or eye. Foreign bodies can be readily located and the removal of thorns, splinters or fragments of grit is made much easier. Ophthalmologists use a refined version of the magnifying glass technically known as a 'loupe'.

5 Patellar hammer This miniature assault-weapon is found in a variety of styles, all designed for a well-aimed blow at the tendon felt just below the front of the knee. This blow sets off an immediate muscular contraction seen as the familiar 'knee jerk'. The whole manoeuvre demonstrates an important reflex circuit.

6 Electric torch If an electric torch is shone in one eye, both pupils can be observed to contract.. The amount of light which enters an eye is regulated by the size of its pupil and in health our two pupils work as a pair. Their co-ordination is complicated and

is controlled by centres deep within the brain. Testing this system is simplicity itself – using the torch as described.

7 Forceps These sophisticated tweezers find their obvious use in removing splinters and surgical stitches. Their great advantage, however, lies in the aseptic dressing of wounds. Forceps are easily sterilized by boiling and, with their aid, wounds can be dressed untouched by bacteria-contaminated human hands.

8 Hypodermic syringe An accepted symbol of the less pleasant side of medicine, the hypodermic syringe is really much maligned. With proper technique, its use for injections or the taking of blood can be quite painless – yet strong men still wilt when faced with it. Unbreakable syringes are available in nylon and disposable injection units are now widely used.

9 Sphygmomanometer This inflatable gauge measures blood pressure. It is wrapped round the upper arm and when pumped up acts as a tourniquet compressing the brachial artery. By listening with a stethoscope as the air is slowly released two pressures can be found. These correspond to the systolic (contraction) and diastolic (relaxation) pressures of the heart.

10 Stethoscope The modern stethoscope – resplendent in chromium and black rubber tubing – conducts sound to both ears simultaneously. Older stethoscopes were made of wood and were designed for one ear only. The obstetric stethoscope, now made in metal, still retains this monaural pattern and appears for all the world like a rose vase from the age of gracious living.

Biblical quiz

The ills of mankind have changed little with the passage of the millenia. Prevention and treatment have made enormous strides yet the disease processes remain remarkably unchanged. Interesting medical conditions can be recognized in the chapters of the Bible and some of these have an extraordinary modern note to them.

The questions of this quiz are linked with the Bible. Can you say...

1 From what did Nebuchadnezzar suffer?

2 What was the treatment given by Elisha to the Shunammite woman's son?

3 How was Eve created?

4 What was the Bible's best advocated tonic?

5 What was the malformation of Moses?

6 What was Sampson's undoing?

7 Why Hannah was deeply depressed?

8 What was Ezekiel's vision.

9 What was Job's malady?

10 From what did St Paul possibly suffer?

answers overleaf

1 Insanity Nebuchadnezzar, creator of the wondrous Hanging Gardens of Babylon, was a military genius and the most powerful of the Babylonian kings. He suffered from psychotic delusions, believing himself to be an animal. He behaved as a beast of the field with nails like birds' talons and eating grass like an ox. His delusions would appear to be symptomatic of severe depressive illness.

2 Mouth-to-mouth breathing Elisha employed mouth–to–mouth breathing when resuscitating the son of the Shunammite woman. In so doing, he anticipated centuries of medical thought which now acclaims this the most efficient means of artificial respiration. Since Elisha's time, colourful resuscitation methods have included rolling the patient over a barrel and even tying him across the back of a galloping horse.

3 Rib transplant The Old Testament describes Eve's creation from one of Adam's ribs. Misrepresentaton of this biblical story later gave rise to a widely held fallacy that men possess fewer ribs than women. This is of course quite untrue. Both man and woman each have twelve pairs of ribs.

4 A merry heart No modern tenets of psychosomatic medicine can better this age-old maxim. Its wisdom is undimmed by the passage of thousands of years. 'Dr Merryman' was long acclaimed the best physician and, of all tonics, joy is still the greatest and most effective known to us.

5 Pair of horns Artistic depiction of Moses with horns growing from his head originates in an early error of biblical translation. This error confused two similar Hebrew words and translated 'his face was horned' in place of 'his face shone'. Michelangelo's famous sculpture of the horned Moses has immortalized this remarkable mistake.

6 A haircut Musclemen appear singularly prone to feminine charm and Samson was no exception. Delilah, extracting the secret of his strength, soon organized an ecclesiastical crew cut. With Samson's hair went Samson's morale, and herein lay the true cause of his ensuing weakness. Myths die hard but abundant hair on body or head is quite unrelated to muscular ability.

7 Infertility With mounting childless years, Hannah became depressed, unable to eat and easily moved to tears – well-known symptoms of a woman deeply disappointed in the hope of motherhood. These symptoms disappeared with the news of her conception and her pregnancy with the infant Samuel. The causes of infertility are complex; solution is frequently to be found in careful medical examination and investigation.

8 Dry bones In Ezekiel's vision, a vast army rose from countless dry and lifeless bones. In life today, by way of contrast, the seeing of visions or hearing of 'voices' is highly suggestive of mental illness and occurs in hallucinatory states. Many would-be prophets since the time of the Bible have in fact suffered from varying forms of schizophrenia.

9 Multiple boils Job erupted in boils from head to toe. His condition – furunculosis – is both demoralizing and extremely painful. It is caused by invading pyogenic bacteria – most notably staphylococci. Job was born ahead of the antibiotic era. He recovered by patience and fortitude, helped little by the comfort of his well-intentioned friends.

10 Epilepsy St Paul's long illness was most probably epilepsy – a disease still little understood even today. Its outward signs range widely from outbursts of explosive behaviour to the full 'grand mal' of the epileptic fit. Their common origin is found in abnormal electrical discharges from the cells of the brain itself. 'Petit mal' or minor epilepsy manifests itself as intermittent 'absences'.

Their claim to fame

Fame, like heaven's rain, falls unabashed on virtue and on vice. A claim to fame need be no claim to merit. Both note and notoriety make equal calls, and infamy in life may often masquerade as fame.

   For better and for worse the persons named here are all famous in medicine. But for what?

1 Hippocrates

2 Baron Münchausen

3 Patrick Bryne

4 René Laënnec

5 Daniel McNaghten

6 Ambroise Paré

7 Burke and Hare

8 Thomas Sydenham

9 Thomas Dover

10 Imhotep

answers overleaf

1 Father of medicine Hippocrates, greatest of all physicians, was born on the Aegean island of Cos in 460 BC It was there that he practised and taught in the open air beneath an enormous plane tree. His clinical methods provided the first realistic basis for medical practice. His famous Oath has set the standard of medical ethics to this present day.

2 Münchausen syndrome Odd individuals present themselves at hospitals with their own requests for immediate admission. An impressive medical history is given and alarming symptoms are described. Later, the whole issue is found to be complete fabrication – but sometimes not before an emergency operation has been performed! This extraordinary condition has become known as Münchausen syndrome, after the genial but irrepressible liar of German fable.

3 Irish giant Bryne (also known as O'Brien) was a famous Irish giant, pursued in life by the eighteenth-century surgeon John Hunter. Hunter wanted Bryne's body for dissection and the Irishman knew it. Bryne made elaborate arrangements for the safety of his body after his death, all of which proved useless. Hunter spent £500 in bribes and obtained the corpse. He later donated Bryne's skeleton to the Royal College of Surgeons.

4 Inventor of the stethoscope René Laënnec, physician to Napoleon, watched two children at play. The one child tapped a wooden log whilst the other listened with an ear placed against the end. Thus was born Laënnec's idea for the first stethoscope – an instrument which opened a new era in diagnosis of diseases of the chest. Laënnec died aged 45 years, himself a victim ironically of tuberculosis of the lung.

5 Criminal responsibility For a defence of insanity, the law requires that an accused person shall not have known what he was doing when committing the crime, or if so, shall not have known he was doing wrong. These are the 'McNaghten Rules', and are named after the mental patient who, in 1843, killed Sir Robert Peel's secretary in mistake for Peel. McNaghten was found insane and was acquitted of murder. A plea of 'diminished responsibility' may now be advanced as a defence.

6 Father of modern surgery The French surgeon Ambroise Paré was born in 1510. Little truth and even less practical value was contained in the armchair type of surgical teaching of his day. Paré, dissatisfied, expressed his disgust and set out for the battlefields. There his observations and his skilful deductions established the foundations of our principles of modern surgery.

7 Resurrection men In the early nineteenth century, Burke and Hare ran a profitable racket robbing graves and supplying Edinburgh Anatomy School with corpses for dissection. Enthusiasm soon outstripped patience and they stepped up trade with a series of murders to obtain further material. When brought to trial, Hare turned King's Evidence. Burke was sentenced and went to the gallows.

8 'English Hippocrates' Disbanded from Cromwell's cavalry at the end of the Civil War, Thomas Sydenham turned to Oxford and studied medicine. He added greatly to our knowledge of fevers and of gout and he re-established the highly important but neglected clinical approach of Hippocrates. St Vitus' dance – a sequel to rheumatic fever – is still called Sydenham's chorea.

9 Robinson Crusoe's rescuer Thomas Dover, pirate no less than physician, rescued Robinson Crusoe (Alexander Selkirk) from his desert island of Juan Fernandez. Like many a member of the sea-going fraternity, Dover had great faith in the therapeutic properties of beer. He freely prescribed this medicinally. His name is found in 'Dover's powder' – a mixture of opium, ipecacuhuana and lactose.

10 Earliest physician Imhotep, the earliest known physician, was an Egyptian vizier. He lived in approximately 3000 BC at the time of the Third Dynasty. No less than his medical skill were his other remarkable abilities as architect, politician, administrator and magician. After his death, Imhotep was deified and worshipped.